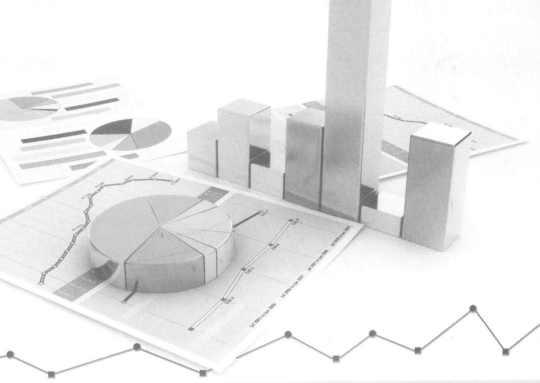

Research
METHODOLOGY
and Basic Biostatistics

RESEARCH METHODOLOGY AND BASIC BIOSTATISTICS

By

Saira Afzal

Mustehsan Bashir

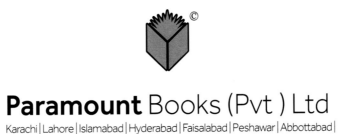

Paramount Books (Pvt) Ltd

Karachi | Lahore | Islamabad | Hyderabad | Faisalabad | Peshawar | Abbottabad |

Paramount Books (Pvt.) Ltd.

152/O, Block-2, P.E.C.H.S., Karachi-75400. Tel: 34310030
Fax: 3455372, E-mail: info@paramountbooks.com.pk
Website: www.paramountbooks.com.pk

ISBN: 978-969-637-083-3

Printed in Pakistan

Contents

To

my teachers, parents, family, friends, students,
educators, and all the researchers of past,
present, and future

Foreword

Rationality and logic are only for those people who apply them. People who create new realities and new logic are beyond these. Let me give you the example of geometry. The shortest path between two points is a straight line (Euclidian geometry) - on a flat paper, but now if you curve this very paper, the straight line you drew is no longer the shortest path between these two points (non-Euclidian geometry). You see, the rules which you considered immutably rational for last two thousand years were in fact just a segment of a bigger reality.

I disagree with the notion of logic and rationality as being the true reflection of what is out there—we must understand that at best our rationality is partial and subjective. You only see part of reality. The remaining "truth" is not available to you.

When you bend the rules of reason and apply it to the domains available to us through traditional rules, new vistas open and a whole new world of ideas becomes available to you and sooner or later these ideas become part of accepted rationality. In fact, these very people who bend the rules of reason, are catalysts for the change of perception and ideas—they are the ones who open new avenues, new realms of reality, and new logic.

For example, if you take into account the randomness at atomic level, there is nothing rational about it. Again, it is considered extremely silly and illogical to ask that what was there before the big bang. This was when something appeared out of nothing. They tell me that this question is considered irrelevant because before the big bang, time was not there. But no matter how I twist it, there is poignant incompleteness in the offered explanation. To satisfy this craving, we came up with this concept of oscillating universe where each expansion is followed by a complete collapse to initiate a new big bang.

This reminds me of a joke. Two Englishmen went to the pub. After consuming pints of lager, flushed and inebriated, they started chatting.

"John, I was wondering last night that if earth is revolving around the sun, then why doesn't it fall down?"

"Pretty relevant question! I was thinking the same. Somebody told me that it is drifting on the back of a big turtle."

"Oh great! But John, what is that great turtle standing on?"

"It is standing on another great turtle."

"And by the way, where is that second turtle standing?"

"Silly, it is turtles all the way down."

Our rationality is like 'turtles all the way down'. We are not looking at the reality of the situation. We are just looking at part of the reality and even that is totally subjective. And then you try to apply this partial knowledge to the whole world. In fact, our partial knowledge will explain only part of reality.

Some apparently frenzied people extend themselves beyond our limits of rationality, explore new avenues and open up a chink for us to see a small new segment of reality. We call their ideas .weird (being afraid of calling "them" weird) only to accept these later, or, sometimes, incarcerate those people in mental asylums or condemn them like Galileo while alive, only to applaud them and cherish their creations after they die.

Have you ever thought about infinity? What is the concept of infinity? The concept is totally incomprehensible beyond imagination. Still, we use it so often without a second thought. Is that symbol for infinity, which you use so conveniently, rational? It is totally irrational, but it does not mean that infinity does not exist. It basically means that at the moment it is beyond my subjective comprehension.

I translate a Persian verse here as you achieve perfection in any task you perform so the world admires you. "Don't undertake an endeavor because it is easy, but do it with a conviction that no one can do it better than you. There is a state called passion which overwhelms all other states of mind."

Professor Faisal Masud
Vice Chancellor
King Edward Medical University
Lahore

Preface

Medicine is the science and art of healing. It encompasses a variety of healthcare practices that have evolved to maintain and restore health. All human societies have beliefs that provide explanations for birth, death, and disease.

Organizing scientific information and writing a book is extremely challenging. To accomplish this task, I was inspired by my teachers, their depth of knowledge, and their remarkably simple ways of teaching. The journey to complete my publication was filled with constant effort, creativity, organizing of scientific truths, overcoming obstacles, and sudden challenges.

> Words come and words go,
>
> But all that an author avows,
>
> Is to bear the trust,
>
> And scribble the truth,
>
> Though it costs much but is worth everything.

Finally I want to acknowledge and mention those people who made this possible. They are my family who stood by me through thick and thin; my teachers who inspired me; and my students who motivated me to accomplish this great task. We are grateful to the World Health Organization for training and research material. We are thankful to all those who extended their help.

Saira Afzal
MBBS, MCPS, MPhil, FCPS

Mustehsan Bashir
MBBS, MCPS
FCPS (Plastic Surgery)

Chapter 1

RESEARCH METHODOLOGY

DEFINITION

An investigation undertaken in order to discover new facts or to get additional information (Oxford Dictionary).

INTRODUCTION TO RESEARCH

- Research is a systematic quest for undiscovered truth.
- Research is an innovative way of thinking.
- Research is the way to solve the problems to decrease human suffering and improve knowledge.

In scientific terms

Research is a systematic, data based, critical and scientific inquiry into a specific problem, undertaken with the objective of finding answers/solutions to it (Fig.1.1).

The main ingredients of research are

- Curiosity to know more
- Objectivity
- Positivity of purpose
- Precision and validity
- Honesty and rigor
- Reproducibility
- Reliability
- Logical reasoning
- Simplicity in explanation

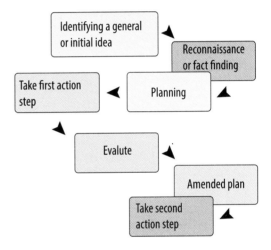

Fig.1.1   Introduction to research

Health research can be divided into two major types:

1. **Basic research** when some new knowledge/technology is generated to deal with health problems.
2. **Applied research** is necessary to identify priority problems and to design and evaluate policies and programs that will deliver the greatest health benefit, making optimal use of available resources and knowledge.

To achieve health for all, necessary planning requires detailed and accurate information/situation analysis regarding needs, priorities, resources, options, cost effectiveness, sustainability and impact (Fig.1.2).

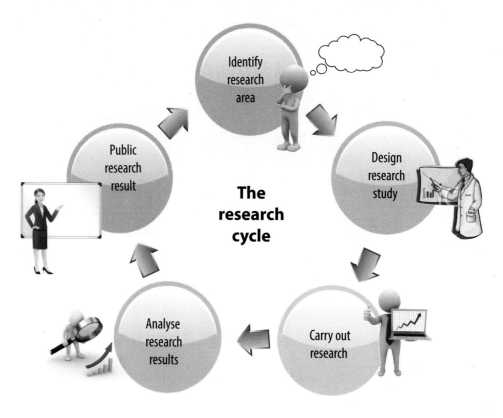

Fig.1.2   The research cycle

There are many terms that are used in research. Examples are discussed below.

Quantitative research

Quantitative research is used to determine the relationship between variables or explore differences between two or more groups.

- It involves the collection and analysis of objective data, often in numerical form.

- Research design and methods are determined prior to the start of data collection and are not flexible

Quantitative research is generally made using scientific methods, which can include:

1. The formulation of hypotheses, theories and models

2. The development of tools and methods for measurement

3. Experimental control and manipulation

4. Collection and analysis of data

5. Modeling and interpretation of data

Although quantitative investigation of the world has existed since people first began to record events or objects that had been counted, the modern idea of quantitative processes have revolutionized research. Quantitative research emphasized the use of the scientific method through observation to empirically test hypotheses explaining and predicting what, where, why, how, and when phenomena occurred. Comte believed only scientific methods rather than previous spiritual explanations for human behavior

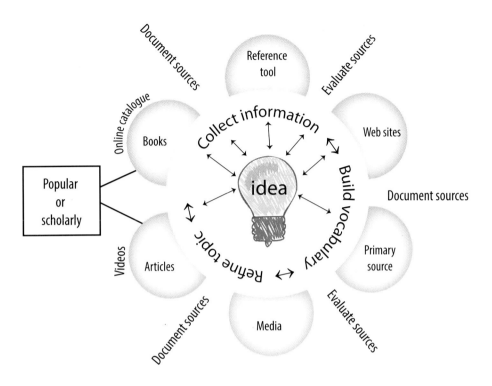

Fig.1.3   Literature search

could advance (Fig.1.3). The theories are put forward in qualitative research and they can be tested before and after applications through quantitative research.

Biostatistics in quantitative research

Statistics is the most widely used branch of mathematics in quantitative research. Quantitative research using statistical methods starts with the collection of data, based on the hypothesis or theory. Usually a big sample of data is collected—this would require verification, validation and recording before the analysis can take place. Software packages such as SPSS and SAS are typically used for this purpose. Causal relationships are studied by manipulating factors thought to influence the phenomena of interest while controlling other variables relevant to the experimental outcomes. In the field of medicine, for example, researchers might measure and study the relationship between dietary fibre intake and measurable physiological effects such as weight loss, controlling for other key variables such as exercise and disease. Quantitatively based opinion surveys are widely used in public health awareness, with statistics such as the proportion of respondents in favor of fast food diet and their body mass indices for obesity. In opinion surveys, respondents are asked a set of structured questions and their responses are tabulated. In the field of science, researchers compile and compare statistics such as temperature or precipitation rates with asthma and allergies over a certain period of time.

Empirical relationships and associations are

also frequently studied by using some form of general linear model, non-linear model, or by using factor analysis. A fundamental principle in quantitative research is that correlation does not imply causation. However, Clive Granger has suggested that a series of co-relations can imply a degree of causality. This principle follows from the fact that it is always possible that a spurious relationship exists for variables between which co-variance is found to some degree. Associations may be examined between any combination of continuous and categorical variables using methods of statistics like correlation and regression analysis.

Role of measurements

The measurements in quantitative research are of two types:

1. Deterministic measurements
2. Probabilistic measurements

Measurement is often regarded as a means by which observations are expressed numerically in order to investigate causal relations or associations. However, it has been argued that measurement often plays a more important role in quantitative research.

Quantitative research may involve the use of *proxies* as stand-ins for other quantities that cannot be directly measured. Tree-ring width, for example, is considered a reliable proxy of ambient environmental conditions such as the warmth of growing seasons or amount of rainfall. Although scientists cannot directly measure the temperature of past years, tree-ring width and other climate proxies have been used to provide a semi-quantitative record of average temperature in the Northern Hemisphere back to 1000 A.D. When used in this way, the proxy record (e.g. tree ring width) only reconstructs a certain amount of the variance of the original record. The proxy may be calibrated (for example, during the period of the instrumental record) to determine how much variation is captured, including whether

both short and long term variation is revealed. In the case of tree-ring width, different species in different places may show more or less sensitivity to, rainfall or temperature: when reconstructing a temperature record there is considerable skill in selecting proxies that are well correlated with the desired variable.

Mixed method research

In most physical and biological sciences, the quantitative or qualitative method is used when appropriate. The majority tendency throughout the history of social science, however, is to use approaches by combining both methods. Qualitative methods might be used to understand the meaning of the conclusions produced by quantitative methods. Using quantitative methods, it is possible to give precise and testable expression to qualitative ideas. This combination of quantitative and qualitative data gathering is often referred to as mixed-methods research. The qualitative research helps to explore ideas, beliefs, myths, theories, cultural influences, mind sets, geographical diversities and effects of implementation of new technologies for better services.

Examples of quantitative research

- Research that consists of the prevalence of polycystic ovarian disease in adolescent females.

- Survey that concludes that the average patient has to wait two hours in the waiting room of a doctor before being examined.

- An experiment in which group x was given two tablets of a drug a day and group y was given two tablets of a placebo a day where each participant is randomly assigned to one or other of the groups. The numerical factors such as two tablets, percentage of elements and the time of drug intake, duration of treatment, days in hospital make the results quantitative.

Qualitative research

Qualitative research is carried out by different methods including interviews, focus group discussions, observations and reflection field notes, various texts, pictures, and other materials. Qualitative research explores ideas, myths, cultural influences, geographical diversities etc.

Characteristics of qualitative research

- Diversity in research design, researcher roles, and data gathering techniques
- Requires the use of a rigorous systematic scientific process
- Data, usually in the form of words (rather than numbers) are detailed, often including description and direct quotations
- Small number of purposefully selected participants or 'cases'
- Used to explore behaviours, moral values, attitudes, opinions, feelings, and social relations of individuals
- Concerned with individuals' perceptions of specific topics, issues, or situations and the meaning they assign to their lives
- Important for theory generation, policy development, improving educational practice, justifying change or a particular practice, and illuminating social issues
- Results are descriptive rather than predictive

Qualitative research often categorizes data into patterns as the primary basis for organizing and reporting results.

Qualitative proposal outline

- Rationale
- Data collection
- Data analysis
- Trustworthiness
- Participants

Qualitative sub-sections of proposal

Qualitative researchers typically rely on the following methods for gathering information:

1. Participant observation
2. Non-participant observation
3. Field notes
4. Reflexive journals
5. Structured interview
6. Semi-structured interview
7. Unstructured interview
8. Analysis of documents and materials
9. Review of historical records

The ways of participating and observing can vary widely from setting to setting. Participant observation is a strategy of reflexive learning, not a single method of observing. In participant observation researchers become members of a culture, group, or setting, and adopt roles to conform to that setting. The aim is for the researcher to gain a closer insight into the culture's practices, motivations and emotions. The researchers' ability to understand the experiences of the culture may be inhibited if they observe without participating. E.g. pediatrician advised Kangaroo care for children after qualitative research in medicine. The researcher spent his time in Africa and observed that children were carried by the mothers mostly in bounded forms like Kangaroo holding their offspring. That bounded infant care provided more secure environment for the children to grow into healthy individuals and helped in developing strong affiliations with their parents.

The obtained data is streamlined to a definite theme or pattern. This is further worked on and alternative research hypothesis is generated which finally provides the basis of the research statement. This will provide

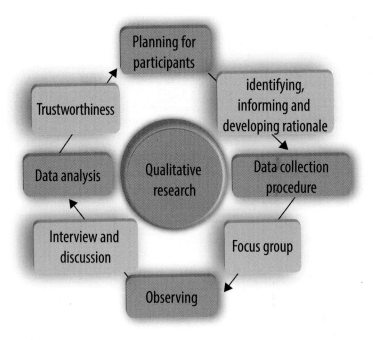

Fig.1.4   Quantitative research

real insight in advantages, disadvantages, acceptance or rejection of new technologies in community settings.

Some distinctive qualitative methods are the use of focus groups and key informant interviews. The focus group technique involves a moderator facilitating a small group discussion between selected individuals on a particular topic. This is a particularly popular method in qualitative research and testing new initiatives with users and workers. Need assessment plans are important parts of qualitative research (Fig.1.4).

In fields that study households, a much debated topic is whether interviews should be conducted individually or collectively (e.g. as couple interviews, family interviews). One traditional and specialized form of qualitative research is called cognitive testing or pilot testing which is used in the development of quantitative survey items. Survey items

are piloted on study participants to test the reliability and validity of the items.

The most frequently used qualitative research approaches include the following points:

1. **Basic qualitative research**: It involves using an eclectic approach taken up to best match the research question at hand (Fig.1.5).

2. **Ethnographic** research: This method is also called ethnomethodology or methodology of the people. An example of applied ethnographic research is the study of a particular culture and their understanding of the role of a particular disease in their cultural framework. E.g. spread of Syphilis among young adults in Congo and its psychosocial effects on their lives.

3. **Grounded theory**: It is an inductive type of research, based in the observations

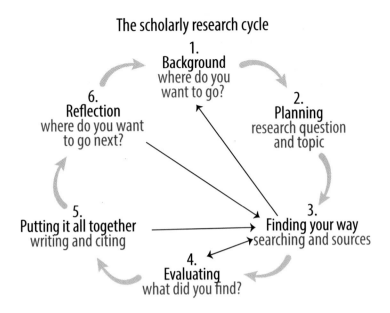

Fig.1.5   The scholarly research cycle

or data from which it was developed; it uses a variety of data sources, including quantitative data, review of records, interviews, observation and surveys.

4. **Phenomenology** describes the subjective reality of an event, as perceived by the study population; it is the study of a phenomenon.

5. **Philosophical research:** It is conducted by field experts within the boundaries of a specific field of study or profession, the best qualified individual in any field of study to use an intellectual analysis, in order to clarify definitions, identify ethics, or make a value judgment concerning an issue in their field of study their lives.

6. **Critical social research:** It is used by a researcher to understand how people communicate and develop symbolic meanings.

7. **Ethical inquiry**: An intellectual analysis of ethical problems. It includes the study of ethics as related to obligation, rights, duty, right and wrong, choice etc.

8. **Foundational research:** Examines the foundations for a science, analyzes the beliefs, and develops ways to specify how a knowledge base should change in light of new information.

9. **Historical research:** Allows one to discuss past and present events in the context of the present condition, and allows one to reflect and provide possible answers to current issues and problems. Historical research helps us in answering questions such as: Where have we come from, where are we, who are we now and where are we going?

10. **Visual methods and photography** for data collection, including photo voice, photo elicitation, collaging, drawing and mapping have been used extensively as a

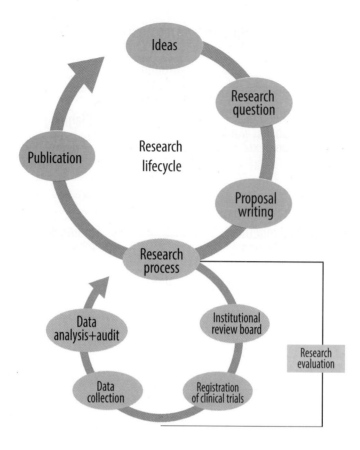

Fig.1.6   Visual methods of research and research cycle

participatory qualitative technique and to make the familiar strange (Fig.1.6).

Data collection and analysis

Data collection

- Preferable to understand the data, adds flexibility to the research
- Typically time-consuming and laborious
- Data collection process emergent and flexible

Data analysis

- Data collection and analysis are conducted simultaneously.

- Data analysis is an on-going process that begins with the first piece of data collected.

- Analysis consists of data management, reduction and coding.

- Goal is to identify patterns (themes) in the data and links between them.

- Software can help to manage data.

Interpretive techniques

The most common analysis of qualitative data is observer impression. That is, expert or bystander observers examine the data, interpret it via forming an impression and report their impression in a structured and sometimes quantitative form.

Coding

Coding is an interpretive technique that both, organizes the data and provides a means to introduce the interpretations of it into certain quantitative methods. Coding helps to change qualitative research into quantitative research. Most coding requires the analyst to read the data and demarcate segments within it, which may be done at different times throughout the process. Each segment is labeled with a code – usually a word or short phrase that suggests how the associated data segments inform the research objectives. Coding may cause loss of richness in data. When coding is complete, the analyst prepares reports by summarizing the prevalence of codes, discussing similarities and differences in related codes across distinct original sources and contexts, or comparing the relationship between one or more codes.

Some qualitative data that is highly structured (e.g. close-end responses from surveys or tightly defined interview questions) is typically coded without additional segmenting of the content. In these cases, codes are often applied as a layer on top of the data. Quantitative analysis of these codes is an analytical step for this type of qualitative data.

Contemporary qualitative data analyses are sometimes supported by computer programs, termed Computer Assisted Qualitative Data Analysis Software. These programs do not change the interpretive nature of coding but rather are aimed at enhancing the analyst's efficiency at data storage/retrieval and at applying the codes to the data. Many programs offer efficiencies in editing and revising coding, which allow for work sharing, peer review, and recursive examination of data.

A disadvantage of the coding method is that it transforms qualitative data into empirically valid data, which contain: actual value range, structural proportion, contrast ratios, and scientific objective properties; thereby draining the data of its variety, richness, and individual character. Analysts removed this limitation by expositing their definitions of codes and linking those codes soundly to the underlying data, thus bringing back some of the variations that might be absent from a mere list of codes.

Summarization of qualitative research

Some qualitative datasets are analyzed without coding. The datasets are summarized and this method is called recursive abstraction. The initial datasets are summarized; those summaries are then further summarized and so on. The end result is a more compact summary with potential of generating a better idea or conclusion.

A limitation of recursive abstraction is that the final conclusions are several times revised and rearranged from the initial data. The main disadvantage is that poor initial summaries will certainly yield an inaccurate final report. This problem is responded by qualitative analysts. They use a coding method and by documenting the reasoning behind each summary step. They cite examples from the data where statements are included and where statements are excluded from the intermediate summary. That explanation at each step would allow better conclusions in the end.

Mechanical techniques

Some techniques rely on using computers to scan and reduce large sets of qualitative data. At their most basic level, mechanical techniques rely on counting words, phrases, or coincidences of tokens within the data. Often referred to as content analysis, the output from these techniques is amenable to many advanced statistical analyses.

Mechanical techniques are particularly well-suited for a few scenarios. One such scenario is for datasets that are simply too large for a human to effectively analyze, or where analysis of them would be costly; relative to the value of information they contain. The cost benefit analysis is causing limitations. Another scenario is when the value of a dataset is the extent to which it contains alarming signs e.g. searching for reports of certain adverse events within a lengthy journal dataset from patients in a clinical trial. The data set may involve positive influences e.g. searching for mentions of new medicine in positive reviews of improving outcomes.

A frequent criticism of mechanical techniques is the absence of a human interpreter. And while masters of these methods are able to write sophisticated software to mimic some human decisions, the most of the analysis is computer based. Analysts responded to these limitations by proving the value of their methods relative to training a human team to analyze the data. The results of qualitative research have reached better conclusions by mechanical data analysis.

Narrative qualitative research

Qualitative research in the last ten years has been characterized by concern with everyday categorization and ordinary storytelling. This "narrative turn" is producing an enormous literature as researchers present sensitizing concepts and perspectives that bear especially on narrative practice, which centers on the circumstances and communicative actions of storytelling. Catherine Riessman (1993) and Gubrium and Holstein (2009) provide analytic strategies, and Holstein and Gubrium (2012) present the variety of approaches in recent comprehensive texts. Relatedly, narrative practice increasingly takes up the institutional conditioning of narrative practice (see Gubrium and Holstein 2000). For example the narrative research on circumcision in decreasing sexually transmitted diseases in Sudan has described the advantages and disadvantages of the procedure for a long period of time.

Dependability

A central issue in qualitative research is trustworthiness (also known as credibility and/or dependability). There are many different ways of establishing trustworthiness, including: member check, interviewer corroboration, peer debriefing, prolonged engagement, negative case analysis, auditability, confirmability. Most of these methods are described by Lincoln and Guba (1985). In quantitative research validity plays a similar role as dependability in qualitative research.

Academic research

By the end of the 1970s, many leading journals began to publish qualitative research articles and several new journals emerged which published only qualitative research studies and articles about qualitative research methods. In the 1980s and 1990s, the new qualitative research journals became more multidisciplinary in focus moving beyond qualitative research disciplinary roots of anthropology, sociology, public health, psychology and philosophy.

Wilhelm Wundt, the founder of scientific psychology, was one of the first psychologists to conduct qualitative research as part of his series of experiments. Early examples of his qualitative research were published in 1900, through 1920, in his 10-volume study, *Völkerpsychologie* (translated to: Social Psychology). Wundt advocated the strong relation between psychology and philosophy. He proposed that there was a gap between psychology and quantitative research that could only be filled by conducting qualitative research. Qualitative researchers dig deep into aspects of human life that could not adequately be covered by quantitative research; aspects such as culture, expression, beliefs, morality and imagination. He provided the comprehensive definitions of qualitative research. The excitement about the groundbreaking form of research was short-lived since many of the pioneering studies with qualitative research had already been conducted. This left many psychologists without the recognition they deserved for their significant work in the field of research. The most important part of qualitative research is need assessment.

Need assessment in qualitative research

The need assessment in qualitative research involves following research methods:

- Using available information in prospective studies
- Observing
- Interviewing
- Administering questionnaire
- Focus group discussion (FGD)
- Nominal group technique (NGT)
- Delphi technique

Focus group discussion (FGD)

- It is a discussion of 6–12 persons guided by a facilitator, during which group members talk freely and spontaneously about a certain topic.
- The purpose of FGD is to obtain in-depth information on concepts, perceptions, and ideas of the group. An FGD aims to be more than a question answer interaction. The idea is that group members discuss the topic among themselves.
- Helps to develop research hypotheses by exploring in greater depth the problem to be investigated and its possible causes.
- Formulate appropriate questions for more structured, larger-scale surveys.
- Supplement information on community knowledge, beliefs, attitude and behavior already available but incomplete or unclear.

- Develop appropriate messages for health education programs.
- Explore controversial topics.

Nominal group technique

- The nominal group technique (NGT) is a technique that is useful when one wants to obtain a consensus on a topic where decision-making can be usefully guided by the perceptions and opinions of the various group members.
- The sequences of the group discussion is usually individual expression followed by "voting" followed by further discussion and another round of voting.
- The group discussion comes to an end when the results of the last vote are not appreciably different from the last-but-one vote.

Delphi technique

The delphi technique and the nominal group technique are used in a situation where a group needs censuses over an issue that is highly value-laden. The major difference is that in the Delphi Technique, groups do not (usually) meet for discussion, they communicate by means of questionnaires.

Each time a questionnaire circulates, the number of permissible answer is reduced based on the answer in the previous questionnaire. The technique needs ample time and participants must have good written communication skills.

Qualitative researchers are interested in understanding the meaning people have constructed. Qualitative research is an effort to understand situations in their uniqueness as part of a particular context and the interactions there (Patton, 1985). A second characteristic of all forms of qualitative research is that the researcher is the primary instrument for data collection and analysis. A third characteristic

Table 1.1   Difference between qualitative and quantitative research

	Qualitative	Quantitative
Social theory	Action	Structure
Methods	Observation, interview	Experiment, survey
Question	What is x? (classification)	How many xs? (enumeration)
Reasoning	Inductive	Deductive
Sampling	Theoretical	Statistical
Strength	Validity	Reliability

Pope and Mays (1995). Reaching the parts other methods cannot reach: An introduction to qualitative methods in health and health services research. BMU: 311: No. 6996

of qualitative research is that it involves fieldwork. The researcher must go to the people, setting, site, institution, in order to observe behavior in its natural setting. A fourth characteristic of qualitative research is that is uses an inductive research strategy. This type of research builds abstractions, concepts, hypothesis, or theories rather than testing existing theory. A fifth characteristic of qualitative finding is in the form of themes, categories, concepts or tentative hypotheses or theories. The product of a qualitative study is richly descriptive. The qualitative research provides ideas, concepts, and scientific truths that are further explored by quantitative research. Thus, mixed research may lead to better outcome measures. The participants in the study should be informed what the terms of the agreement (consent form) are, and aims and objectives of the research. All personal information should be kept confidential and must tell the truth when a researcher writes up the final report.

Implementation research in situations where information is lacking, or unreliable, decision-making based on assumptions and unjustified conclusions may result in the selection of inappropriate policies and programs, consequences of which are often grave.

Therefore provide reliable and accurate information for suitable decision making and planning.

The importance of research in identifying solutions and options for overcoming implementation obstacles in health systems and programmes is widely recognized. *This form of research addresses implementation bottlenecks, identifies optimal approaches for a particular setting, and promotes the uptake of research findings*: ultimately, it leads to improved health care and its delivery.

While IR has been defined in various ways by different institutions, common interpretations focus on the systematic approach to understanding and addressing barriers to effective and quality implementation of health interventions, strategies and policies. IR is demand-driven and the research questions are framed based on needs identified together with relevant stakeholders/ implementers in the health system. Key characteristics of IR are summarized in Fig.1.7.

The need to address implementation bottlenecks is often greatest in settings where health systems are the weakest or non-existent. Unfortunately, local institutions often have limited knowledge of IR and lack essential capacities to frame relevant research questions, and conduct, manage and interpret research results for programme planning and policy implementation. Academic public health curricula tend not to focus on such research. As a result, most training does not adequately prepare researchers, practitioners, providers or decision-makers for essential partnership and interdisciplinary approaches.

The intervention. The characteristics of the intervention determine whether it will be adopted or 'fit' for the local health system. Here the term 'intervention' includes the core components and those elements that may be adapted to suit local needs and/or conditions. The characteristics of core components, such as complexity, cost and evidence strength, play a crucial role.

Outer setting. This includes the economic, political and social contexts in which an intervention is carried out and that are external to the implementing organization/institution. It is influenced by external policies and incentives—such as global funding streams—as well as by interactions and peer pressure among organizations.

Inner setting. This refers to the context within the implementing organization/institution. It includes the structure of the organization, its culture (internal climate) and networks, as well as readiness for change.

Individuals involved. These are people who have a direct role in the implementation process.

This includes health care providers, managers in various parts of the organization/institution, policy-makers and many other stakeholders and beneficiaries. In addition to the usual concerns regarding the capacity to implement, their perceptions and attitudes towards the intervention have an important influence on their commitment to its success and impact.

Process for implementation. This incorporates all of the methods and approaches used in facilitating adoption of the intervention at all levels of the organization, including the planning of strategies and activities. Processes include both those explicitly planned and unforeseen ones that emerge during implementation.

Advantages of research

- Provides extensive reading to build a sizeable pool of knowledge of different situations and options.

- Provides an opportunity to do significant independent work on a problem /area that will better prepare a professional for achieving identified expertise.

- Provides opportunities to publish one's observations and share knowledge in a scientific manner.

Characteristics of research

- Research demands a clear understanding of the problem and finding research action impact.

- Research builds upon existing data using both positive and negative findings.

- Research collects new information to answer the original research question.

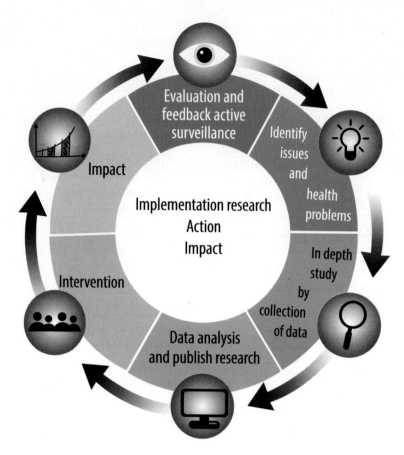

Fig.1.7   Characteristics of implementation research (IR)

OUTLINE OF RESEARCH PROCESS

STEPS IN DESIGNING AND CONDUCTING RESEARCH

- Thinking about a research topic/research question
- Literature search/review
- Formulating a research question/objective
- Matching the Research Design to the research objectives
- Defining and clarifying the research Variables Analysis plan

Research process

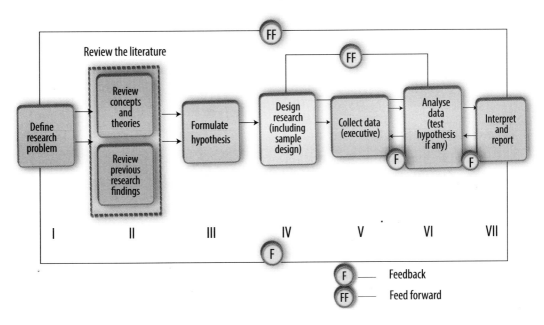

Fig.2.1   Research process

- Drawing the Sample
- Developing the tools and defining the methods of data collection
- Monitoring and carrying out the research
- Preparing the data for Analysis
- Analyzing data
- Writing the research report in the form of an original articlethesis (Fig.2.1).

SELECTING A RESEARCH TOPIC

Criteria for selecting a research topic

- Relevance
- Innovation
- Feasibility
- Acceptability
- Cost-effectiveness
- Ethical consideration
- Evaluation

Relevance

- How big is the problem?
- How important is it to look for relevant solutions to it?
- Are solutions to it available, if so how effective have they been proved?
- Is the problem important in our local set up (Fig.2.3)?

Innovation

- In case the topic has been researched, what new angle are you looking at?
- This should be addressed as the rationale of the study (qualifying the "so what" answer). It should substantially increase the knowledge and should provide with directions to policy formulation (evidence-based)(Fig.2.4).

Feasibility

Consider the resources that are required to carry out the project.

Acceptability

Research a topic which has the interest and support of the authorities.

Cost-effectiveness

Whether the resources of

- Time
- Money
- Manpower

Being invested in the study are worthwhile (Table 2.1)

Ethical consideration

- Cultural sensitivity must be given careful consideration.
- Informed consent must be ensured.
- Will treatment be given to individuals identified during study who require treatment?

Rating scale

1. = Low
2. = Medium
3. = High
- Total Score out of 18

Proposed Topic

Relevance 1, 2, 3

Innovation 1, 2, 3

Feasibility 1, 2, 3

Acceptability 1, 2, 3

Cost Effectiveness 1, 2, 3

Ethical issues 1, 2, 3

Potential research questions arise from day to day clinical practice.

Table 2.1   Selecting a research topic

Issue	Question
Abnormality	Is the patient sick or well?
Diagnosis	How accurate are tests used to diagnose?
Frequency	How often does a disease occur?
Risk	What factors are associated with an increased risk of disease?
Prognosis	What are the consequences of having a disease?
Treatment	How does treatment change the course of disease?
Prevention	Does an intervention on well people keep disease from arising?
	Does early detection and treatment improve the course of disease?
Cause	What conditions lead to disease?
	What are the pathogenetic mechanisms of disease?
Cost	How much will care for and illness cost?

Research begins with a problem.

- This problem need not be earth-shaking.

Identifying this problem can actually be the hardest part of research. In general, good research projects should:

- Address an important question.
- Advance knowledge.

Sources of Research Problems:

- Observation
- Literature reviews
- Professional conferences
- Experts

Literature review

This step is an essential preliminary task in order to find out about an available body of knowledge in your interest area. In addition, literature review is an integral part of the entire research process and makes valuable contribution to every operational step. Reviewing literature can be time consuming, daunting and frustrating, but is also rewarding.

Its functions are:

1. to keep up with the latest developments in your field,

2. to understand your topic in the context of what is already known,

3. to document important facts and ideas you wish to research in the light of previous work done on it, and

4. to avoid rediscovering the truth.

5. this helps in bringing clarity and focus to the research problem and improving the study methodology. Above all, it broadens the investigator's knowledge.

Search strategy on internet

- Summarize your topic in one or two sentences.
- Identify the unique ideas or concepts associated with your topic.
- Choose appropriate keywords for each concept.
- Establish the relationship between each keyword and the concept.
- Choose a bibliographic database.

Actually there are many online medical databases:

- MedLine (OVID): http://gateway.ovid.com
- Mdconsult: http:// home.mdconsult.com
- HINARI: http:// www.who.int/hinari/usinghinari/en/index.html

- PubMed: http:// www.ncbi.nlm.gov./ pubmed

- And many others

For an academic paper, you should use books and articles as well as websites that collect important information on your topic. During the literature review, the investigator can note the detailed description of methodologies and instruments used in previous research. In addition these detailed descriptions are the best way to determine possible approaches appropriate to their needs, such as sampling techniques, interviewing, data collection methods, and interventions (Fig.2.2).

Formulating research objective

"A question well asked is a question half answered":. The way the question is stated shows what data will be necessary to answer (or test) it, and probably suggests also how and from where or from whom the data will be obtained. This brings us to research objectives.

Objectives are defined as: an intent, communicated by a statement describing the plan of the researcher in clear, measurable terms.

Importance of research objectives:

- Brings focus to the study

- Avoids collection of unnecessary data

- Determines an appropriate study design

- Helps determine analysis plan

The objective should be "SMART"

- S: Specific

- M: Measureable

- A: Achievable

- R: Reproducible

- T: Time bound

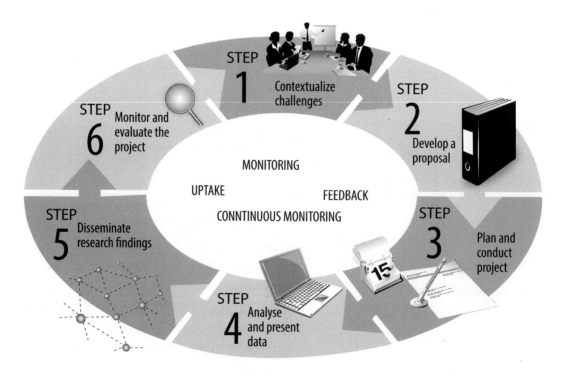

Fig.2.2   Summary of methodologies and approaches

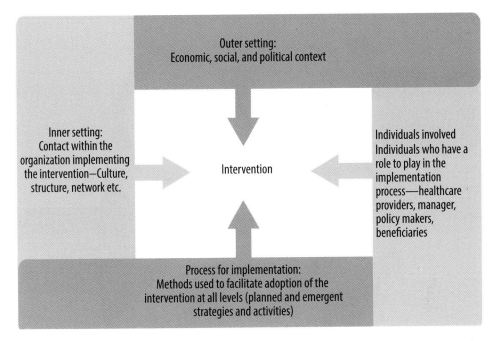

Fig.2.3   Interventional research—relevance

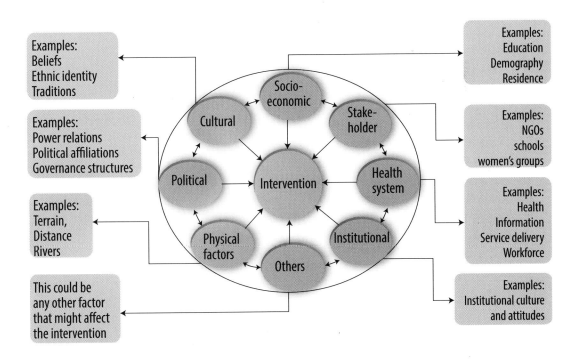

Fig.2.4   Interventional research—innovation

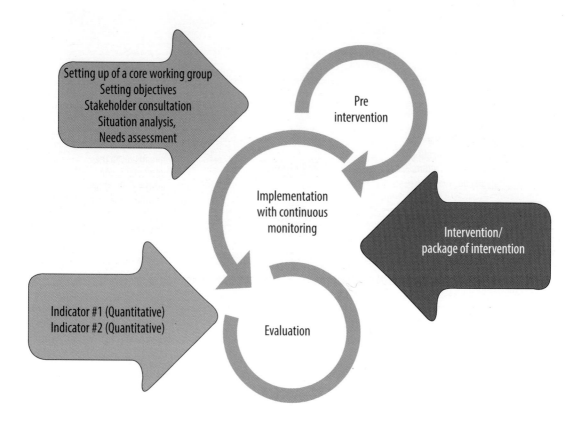

Fig.2.5   Interventional research and evaluation

Examples

1. To determine the frequency of anaemia in pregnant women visiting tertiary care facilities of the punjab

2. To determine association between maternal smoking and low birth weight

3. To compare the effectiveness of dressing A vs. dressing B in patients presenting with infected wounds of the foot

Operational definition

Define each technical term as it is used in relation to your research project. This helps remove significant ambiguity from the research itself by ensuring that reviewers, while they may not agree with your definitions, at least know what you're talking about. Thus operational definition is the definition of the exposure and outcome variables of interest in context to objectives in a particular study and their means of measurement/determination. For example, anaemia, maternal smoking, low birth weight, effectiveness, wound healing.

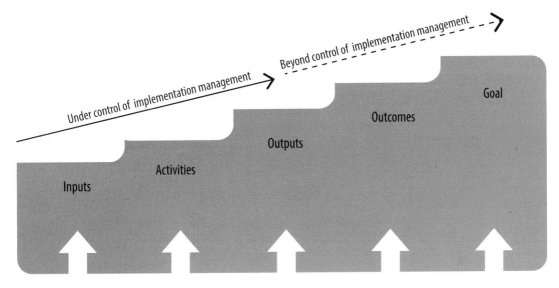

Fig.2.6   Monitoring and evaluation in research

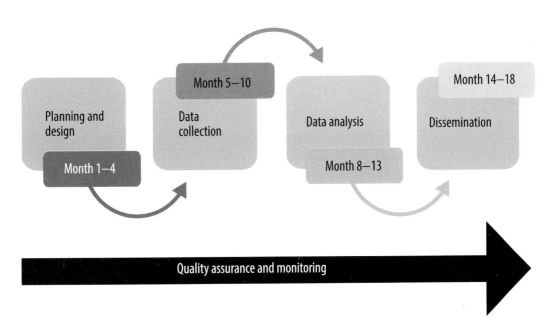

Fig.2.7   Evaluation and monitoring of research

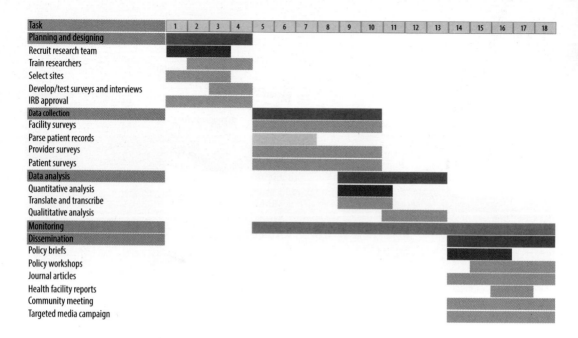

Fig.2.8   Time frame for research activities

Chapter

3 STUDY DESIGNS

Depending on the existing state of knowledge about a problem that is being studied, a different type of study design may be chosen and it depends on:

1. The type of problem
2. The knowledge already available about the problem
3. The resources available for the study

When exploring more complicated management problems and many health problems, we usually want to go further and determine the extent to which one or several variables contribute to the problem. For example, to find out the profile/characteristics of the patients suffering from an epidemic of influenza, we may need a simple descriptive study, whereas to study the contribution of a low-fibre diet to cancer of the large intestine, we will need more rigorous analytical or experimental studies before we decide on appropriate interventions.

Several classifications of study types are available in medical literature. There is an array of different terminologies, at times causing considerable confusion. The classification given in this text is the one suggested by the World Health Organization.

The research studies are first classified on the basis of **intervention**. If the researcher just describes and analyzes researchable objects or situations but does **not** intervene, it is called a *Non-interventional* or *Observational*

Study. If the researcher **manipulates objects** or **situations** and measures the outcome of his manipulation (*e.g.* by implementing intensive health education and measuring the improvement in immunization rates), it is called *Interventional* or *experimental study.*

NON-INTERVENTIONAL OR OBSERVATIONAL STUDIES

Non-interventional studies are further divided into the following two categories: Descriptive studies and analytical studies.

Descriptive studies

Descriptive studies involve the systematic collection and presentation of data to give a clear picture of a particular situation. Descriptive studies can be carried out on a small or large scale.

Descriptive case studies describe in-depth the characteristics of one or a limited number of "cases." A case may be, for example, a patient, a health centre, or a village. Such a study can provide useful insight into a problem.

Case studies are common in social sciences, management sciences, and clinical medicine. For example, in clinical medicine the characteristics of a hitherto unrecognized illness may be documented as a case study. This is often the first step towards building up a clinical picture of that illness.

However, if one wishes to test whether the findings pertain to a larger population or not, an extensive cross sectional survey has to be designed.

Analytical studies

An analytical study attempts to establish association or risk factors for certain problems. This is done by comparing two or more groups, some of which have or develop the problem and some of which have not.

Three commonly used types of analytical studies are discussed here.

1. Cross-sectional studies
2. Case-control studies
3. Cohort studies

CROSS-SECTIONAL STUDIES

Cross-sectional surveys focus on comparing as well as describing groups.

Cross sectional studies aim at quantifying the distribution of certain variables in a study population at a point of time. They may cover, for example:

- Physical characteristics of people, materials, or the environment, as in prevalence surveys
- Evaluation of coverage of immunization etc.
- The knowledge, attitudes, beliefs, and opinions of people, that may help to explain that behaviour (KAP studies), or events that occurred in the population

These studies quantify the burden of disease in a given population and are useful for hypothesis generation (Fig.3.1).

Cross-sectional surveys cover a sample of the population. If a cross-sectional study covers the total population, it is called a **census.**

The outcome measure of a cross sectional study could be point prevalence/period prevalence.

The findings are usually presented as proportions.

Example1

To compare two teaching methods—lectures vs. small group discussions for better learning outcomes among students in University XYZ. A survey on teaching methods may wish to establish the following through data analysis:

1. The distribution of demographic variables among students in two groups.
2. The level of satisfaction and improving knowledge from certain baseline measures in two groups of students.
3. The statistical significance of better class results in one group of students as compared to others.

Example 2

To compare malnutrition among school children aged 10–16 years in an urban community. A survey on malnutrition may wish to establish the following through data analysis:

1. The percentage of malnourished children in a certain population
2. The age and gender distribution with certain parameters of malnutrition
3. Socioeconomic, physical, political and demographic variables that influence the availability of food feeding practices
4. The knowledge, beliefs, and opinions that influence these practices

Example 3

A cross—sectional study of breast feeding practices and prevention of obesity in children and adults. It will highlight the following points.

- Obesity is the most frequent nutritional

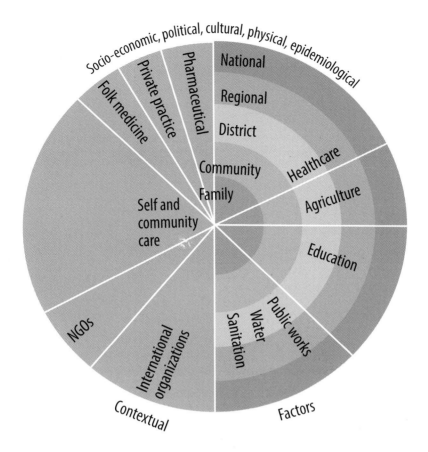

Fig.3.1   Community research—cross-sectional model

disorder in children, and is an important risk factor for cardiovascular disease in adulthood.

- Preventing obesity should be a useful strategy in preventing later heart diseases in adults because weight loss interventions in obese children are costly and rarely successful.

- Data from a cross—sectional study in Bavaria suggested that the risk of obesity in children at the time of school entry can be reduced by breast feeding: A 35% reduction occurs if children are breastfed for 3 to five months.

- Preventing obesity and its consequences

may be an important argument in the drive to encourage breast feeding practices in industrialized countries.

Example 4

To compare the immunization status among children in an urban community. A survey on immunization may help to establish the following through data analysis.

1. The percentage of immunization children in a certain population

2. The age, gender and geographical distribution of immunized children in urban community

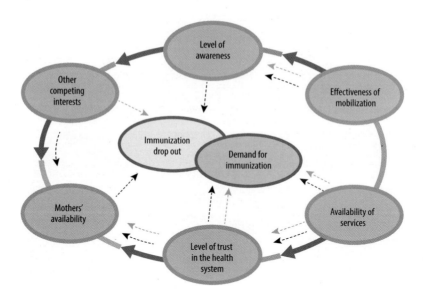

Fig.3.2   Cross-sectional study to determine immunization practice

3. Socio-economic, geographical, political, and demographical variables that influence the immunization practices (Fig.3.2)

CASE CONTROL STUDIES

*   Observational study in which both exposure and outcome (disease) have occurred before the start of the study
*   Involves two populations—cases and controls
*   Cases are subjects who have the disease while controls are free from the disease but are otherwise similar to cases regarding age, sex, occupation, social status etc.
*   Case-control studies often used to identify factors that may have contributed to a medical condition

Example

4. Case control study to find the association of lung cancer with shisha smoking in an adult population

5. Case control study to find the association of deep venous thrombosis with oral contraceptive pills

Basic steps in conducting a case control study

1. Selection of cases and controls
2. Matching
3. Measurement of exposure
4. Analysis and interpretation

1. Selection of cases

A. Definition of a case is crucial and involves:

    i. Diagnostic criteria: Should be well defined, measurable, and the same among all the subjects of cases

    ii. Eligibility criteria: Newly diagnosed cases within a specified period of time are usually considered eligible than old cases i.e. cases in advanced stages of the disease (prevalent cases)

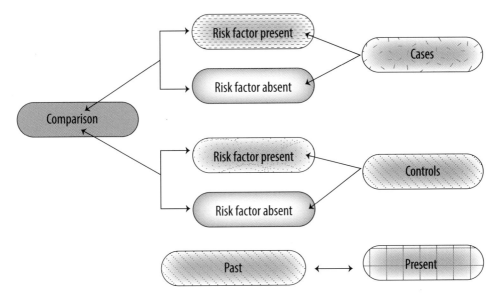

Fig.3.3   Case control study

B. Source of cases:

1. **Hospitals**: Cases drawn from
   - single hospital or
   - a network of hospitals, admitted during a specified period of time

2. **General population**: All cases of the study disease occurring within a defined area during a specified period of time are ascertained, often through a survey or disease registry or hospital network

Selection of controls

- Controls must be free from the disease under study.
- Difficulties arise if the disease is sub-clinical and the diagnosis is difficult.

Sources of controls

1. Hospital controls
2. Relatives
3. Neighbourhood controls
4. General population

How many controls are needed?

If many cases (common problem) = 1:1

If less cases (rare problem) = 1:2, 1:3 or 1:4 controls

2. Matching

Cases and controls must be similar regarding certain pertinent selected variables (e.g. age) that are likely to influence the outcome (confound). However, the variable we wish to measure should not be matched.

Lack of matching could distort or confound the results.

Kinds of matching procedures

1. Assigning cases to strata based on their characteristics (e.g. age, occupation, social class) and then establishing appropriate controls. The frequency distribution of the variable in the study and the control group must be the same

2. Pairs

3. Measurement of exposure

- Definitions and criteria about exposure
- Obtained by interviews, questionnaires, past records (hospital records, employment records)
- Bias occurs if exposure is not measured properly

3. Analysis

To find out:

A. A proportion of exposed among the cases and controls to suspected factor and comparing these proportions by chi-square and controls to a suspected factor

B. Estimation of disease risk associated with exposure (odds ratio)

A. Exposure rates:

A case control study provides a direct estimation of the proportions (frequency of exposure) to a suspected factor in disease and non-disease groups.

Method to calculate exposure

Example: A case control study of smoking and lung cancer.

Table 3.1.   2x2 table to show results

	CA	Healthy
Smoking	a	b
Present	33	55
Absent	c 2	d 27

Cases = $a/(a+c) = 33/35 = 94.2\%$

Controls = $b/(b+d) = 55/82 = 67\%$

$P < 0.001$

(If P-value is< or=0.05), it is regarded as statistically significant. The smaller the P-value, the greater the statistical significance or probability that the association is not due to chance alone.

Limitations of case control study

- It does not provide incidence rates.
- Relative risk cannot be calculated as there is no appropriate denominator.
- Relative Risk can be determined only from a cohort study.

Odds ratio

- Can be derived from a case control study
- Measure of the strength of the association between risk factor and outcome
- Disease under investigation must be rare (chronic diseases)

How to calculate odds ratio

- The cross product of the entries.
- Odds ratio $= ad/bc$.
- Odds ratio $= 33 \times 27/55 \times 2 = 8.1$ times higher

Bias in case control study

- Definition: Bias is any systematic error in the determination of the association between the exposure and the disease.
- Disadvantage: The relative risk estimate may increase or decrease as a result of the bias.

Varieties of bias

1. Bias due to confounding: This can be removed by matching.
2. Memory or recall bias: Cases better recall their past history.
3. Selection bias: Cases and controls may not be representatives of cases and controls in the general population.
4. Berksonian bias: This is caused by different rates of admission to hospitals for people with different diseases.
5. Interviewer's bias: When the interviewer

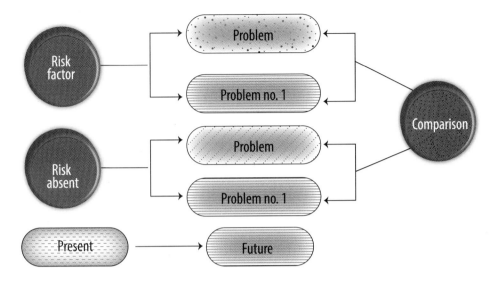

Fig.3.4   Cohort study

knows the hypothesis and also knows who the cases are. This leads him to ask the cases questions more thoroughly. This type of bias can be eliminated by double-blinding.

6. Measurement bias: This occurs when the methods of measurement are dissimilar among groups of patients.

Schematic diagram of case-control study

In case control studies, the direction of our enquiry is from the present to the past. In other words we have the outcome and we are looking for the causes or risk factors. In the example of coronary heart disease, we have the outcome that is coronary heart disease and we are exploring their past to find out the modifiable factors which contributed to the coronary heart disease. In other words our direction of enquiry is backwards. When we look toward the past, this is called **Retrospection**. Therefore sometimes case-control studies are referred to as retrospective studies.

Example

A case control study: Effects of potentially modifiable risk factors associated with myocardial infarction in 52 countries (the INTERHEART study)

More than 80% of the global burden of cardiovascular disease occurs in low-income and middle-income countries, knowledge of the importance of risk factors is largely derived from developed countries. Therefore, the effect of such factors on risk of coronary heart disease in most regions of the world is unknown. Thus, to establish association of risk factors with the risk of coronary heart disease, a case control study was planned.

Methods

The researcher established a standardized case-control study of acute myocardial infarction in 52 countries, representing every inhabited continent. 15,152 cases and 14,820 controls were enrolled. The relation of smoking, history of hypertension or diabetes, waist/hip ratio, dietary patterns, physical activity, consumption of alcohol, blood apolipoproteins (Apo), and psychosocial factors to myocardial infarction were reported. Odds ratios and their 99% CIs for the association of risk factors to myocardial infarction and their population attributable risks (PAR) were calculated.

Findings

The risk factors (independent variables) in the case control study were smoking (odds ratio 2.87 for current *vs* never, PAR 35.7% for current and former *vs* never), raised ApoB/ApoA1 ratio (3.25 for top *vs* lowest quintile, PAR 49.2% for top four quintiles *vs* lowest quintile), history of hypertension (1.91, PAR 17.9%), diabetes (2.37, PAR 9.9%), abdominal obesity (1.12 for top *vs* lowest tertile and 1.62 for middle *vs* lowest tertile, PAR 20.1% for top two tertiles *vs* lowest tertile), psychosocial factors (2.67, PAR 32.5%), daily consumption of fruits and vegetables (0.70, PAR 13.7% for lack of daily consumption), regular alcohol consumption (0.91, PAR 6.7%), and regular physical activity (0.86, PAR 12.2%), were all significantly related to acute myocardial infarction (p<0.0001 for all risk factors and p=0.03 for alcohol). These associations were noted in men and women, old and young, and in all regions of the world. Collectively, these nine risk factors accounted for 90% of the PAR in men and 94% in women.

Interpretation

Abnormal lipids, smoking, hypertension, diabetes, abdominal obesity, psychosocial factors, consumption of fruits, vegetables, and alcohol, and regular physical activity account for most of the risk of myocardial infarction worldwide in both sexes and at all ages in all regions. This finding suggested that approaches to prevention can be based on similar principles worldwide and have the potential to prevent most premature cases of myocardial infarction.

COHORT STUDIES

In a cohort study, a group of individuals that is exposed to a risk factor (study group) is compared with a group of individuals not exposed to the risk factor (control group). The researcher follows both groups over time and compares the occurrence of the problem that he or she expects to be related to the risk factor in the two groups to determine whether a greater proportion of those with the risk factor are indeed affected.

A well known example of a cohort study is the Framingham Study of smokers and nonsmokers that was conducted to determine the importance of smoking as a risk factor for developing lung cancer.

A study may start with one large cohort. After the cohort is selected, the researchers may then determine who is exposed to the risk factor (e.g. smoking) and who is not, and follow the two groups over time to determine whether the two groups develop lung cancer. If it is not possible to select a cohort and divide it into a study group and a control group, two cohorts may be chosen, one in which the risk factor is present (study group) and one in which it is absent (control group). In all other respects the two groups should be as similar as possible. The control group should be selected at the same time as the study group and both should be followed with the same intensity.

Example 1

Researchers were suspecting that bankers were suffering from coronary heart disease (CHD). Now they wanted to be sure about the hypothesis that banking is a risk factor for heart disease. First they selected 100 bankers and then 100 controls who were not bankers, matched on the basis of age and sex and other risk factors. They followed this group of people to see how many got CHD. They found that Out of 100 bankers 60 developed CHD and of the control group, 30 developed CHD.

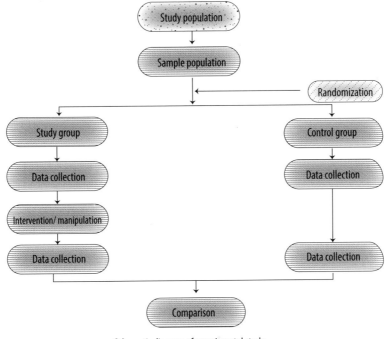

Schematic diagram of experimental study

Fig.3.5   Schematic diagram of experimental study

Schematic diagram of cohort study

In cohort study we start with non-diseased persons. Both groups are free from the disease being studied. One group has the suspected Risk Factor, while the other does not. We look towards the development of disease in both groups. In other words our direction of enquiry is forward i.e., from present to the Future. When we look towards the future, this is called prospection. Therefore, sometimes Cohort studies are also called **Prospective studies.**

Example 2

A cohort study of 22,707 Chinese men in Taïwan was set up to investigate the association between Hepatitis B and the development of Hepatocellular Carcinoma. The study was conducted among male government employees who were enrolled through routine health care services. All participants completed a health questionnaire and provided a blood sample at the time of their entry into the study. Participants were then followed up for an average of 23.3 years and association of Hepatitis B was found significant with Hepatocellular Carcinoma.

(Beasley et al., 1981).

Uses and limitations of different types of analytical studies

Barring certain ethical considerations, you may use any of the three types of analytical studies (cross-sectional, case-control, or cohort) to investigate possible causes of a problem.

Assume there is a causal relationship between the use of a certain water source and the occurrence of diarrhea among children less than five years of age in a village with different water sources.

In a cross-sectional study, you could interview mothers to determine whether their children had diarrhea during, for example, the past month, obtain information on their source of drinking water, and compare the source of drinking water of children who did and did not have diarrhea. The information of disease and possible factors is obtained at the same time.

You can also conduct a case-control study. For example, you may compare children who present themselves at a health centre with diarrhea (cases) during a particular period of time with children presenting themselves without diarrhoea or other disease e.g. coming for immunization (controls) during the same time and determine which source of drinking water they had used. The information on possible exposure to source of drinking water is obtained from history. Here only strength of association can be measured.

You can select a group of children less than five years and classify them based on their exposure to a bad or a safe water supply. Then check at regular intervals (e.g. every week) whether the children have had diarrhea. Children using a suspected source and those using other sources of water supply will be compared with regard to the incidence of diarrhea (cohort study).

Cross-sectional studies and case-control studies are relatively quick and inexpensive to undertake. The major problem with case-control studies is the selection of appropriate control groups. The matching of cases and controls has to be done with care. Another problem with a case control study is the recall bias. People may not remember the past history very accurately.

Cohort studies are a way to establish causal relationships. However, they take longer than case-control studies and are labour intensive and, therefore, expensive. The major problems are usually related to the identification of all cases in a study population and to the inability to follow up all persons included in the study over a number of years because of population movement. Loss to follow up is a serious source of bias in such studies. This is called attrition. If the attrition rate exceeds 15% the cohort study loses its strength. One objection to the cohort study is that the subjects with a risk factor may be basically different (e.g. genetically) than the comparison group.

INTERVENTIONAL OR EXPERIMENTAL STUDIES

In intervention studies, the researcher manipulates a situation by his/her own design and measures the effects of the manipulation. Usually (but not always) two groups are compared, one in which the intervention takes place (e.g. treatment with a new drug) and another group that remains "untouched" (e.g. treatment with a standard drug).

There are two types of intervention studies:

- Experimental studies
- Quasi-experimental studies

Experimental studies

Experimental design is the only type of study design that can actually prove causation. In an experimental study, individuals are randomly allocated to at least two groups. One group is subjected to an intervention or experiment, while the other group(s) is not. The outcome of the intervention is measured by comparing the two groups. The experimental studies are also called **Randomized controlled trials (RCT).**

The classical experimental study design has three characteristics;

- **Randomization:** the researcher takes care to **randomly** assign subjects to either control or experimental groups. "Random" does not mean "at will". It is a scientific process.

- **Control:** the researcher introduces one

or more control group(s) to compare with the experimental group.

- **Manipulation:** the researcher does something different/additional to one group of subjects in the study.

Schematic diagram of experimental study

Quasi-experimental studies

In a quasi-experimental study, at least one characteristic of a true experiment is missing, either randomization or the use of a separate control group. However, a quasi-experimental study always includes manipulation of an independent variable that serves as the intervention.

Most of the quasi-experimental studies uses two (or more) groups, one of, which serves a control group in which no intervention takes place. Both groups are observed before as well as after the intervention, to test if the intervention has made any difference. The subjects in the two groups (study and control groups) have not been randomly assigned.

Examples

1. **Person-by-treatment** designs are the most common type of a quasi experiment design. In this design, the experimenter measures at least one independent variable. Along with measuring one variable, the experimenter will also manipulate a different independent variable. Because there is manipulating and measuring of different independent variables, the research is mostly done in laboratories. An important factor in dealing with person-by-treatment designs are that random assignments will need to be used in order to make sure that the experimenter has complete control over the manipulations that are being done to the study.

   An example of this type of design was performed at the university of notre dame. The study was conducted to see if being mentored for your job led to increased job satisfaction. The results showed that many people who did have a mentor showed very high job satisfaction.

2. **Natural experiments** are a different type of quasi experiment design used by researchers. It differs from person-by-treatment in a way that there is not a variable that is being manipulated by the experimenter. Instead of controlling at least one variable like the person-by-treatment design, experimenters do not use random assignments and leave the experimental control up to chance. The manipulations occur naturally, and although this may seem like an inaccurate technique, it has actually proven to be useful in many cases. These are the studies done to people who had something sudden happen to them. This could mean good or bad, traumatic or euphoric. An example of this could be studies done on those who have been in a car accident and those who have not. Car accidents occur naturally, so it would not be ethical to stage experiments to traumatize subjects in the study. These naturally occurring events have proven to be useful for studying post traumatic stress disorder cases.

3. **Ecological studies** are quasi experiment studies to compare the outcome of disease in particular geographical settings. An example of an ecologic study is one of the associations between increasing primary care physician supply and the incidence and mortality rates for colorectal cancer in 67 Florida counties. They found a strong negative correlation between primary care physician supply and both incidence (-0.46) and mortality (-0.29). That is, having a greater proportion of primary care physicians in a county was associated with a reduction in the incidence and mortality due to colorectal cancer.

Hybrid study designs

it is sometimes expedient to include a case-control design within a retrospective or a prospective cohort study. Suppose that an investigator is interested in whether serum beta-carotene affects the risk of colon cancer. In a traditional prospective cohort study, beta carotene levels would be measured in blood samples from all the cohort members, and subsequent disease incidence would be determined according to the level of beta-carotene. In a nested case control study, blood samples from all of the (say, 10,000) cohort members would be frozen and stored without measuring beta-carotene. Suppose that after 10 years, 200 cohort members had been diagnosed with colon cancer and 9,800 are free of colon cancer. All of the cases and a sample of, for example, 400 controls without the disease could be selected and beta-carotene could be measured in the stored serum. The cases and controls could then be compared according to beta-carotene level, as in a traditional case-control study. Controls are usually selected from unaffected cohort members who are still alive and under surveillance at the time the cases developed the disease. Typically the controls are matched to the cases according to age, gender, and time of entry into the cohort. Sampling non-diseased individuals greatly reduces the cost compared with measurement of beta-carotene levels of all 10,000 cohort members but assures that beta-carotene measures represent levels before the diagnosis of the disease. The availability of a variety of banks of stored blood and the current interest in serologic and genetic predictors of disease make nested case-control studies an attractive approach, as long as the marker of interest does not undergo degradation over time and the specimens have been processed in a way that allows the marker to be determined in the sample.

A case-cohort study is another method of increasing efficiency compared to traditional cohort studies. Like the nested case-control study, all cases and a sample of controls are included, but the controls are sampled from the entire cohort, including cases of other diseases, and are not matched to the cases. Instead, other relevant variables are taken into account in the statistical analysis. A case-cohort design is particularly useful when the associations between an exposure (e.g. serum beta-carotene) and several diseases (e.g. cancers of the colon, lung, and pancreas) are of interest. Nested case-control and case-cohort designs are also particularly useful when collecting information about confounders from a cohort involves review of medical records or a survey. In these instances, data can be collected from all of the cases and a sample of controls, greatly reducing the cost of data collection.

Clinical trials

1. A clinical trial is a research study to answer specific questions about new therapies or vaccines or new ways of using known treatment.

2. Clinical trials are used to determine whether new drugs or treatment are both safe and effective.

3. Carefully conducted clinical trials are the fastest and safest way to find treatments that work.

In phase I clinical trials, researchers test a new drug or treatment in a small group of people (20 – 80) for the first time to evaluate its safety, determine a safe dosage range, and identify side effects.

In phase II clinical trials, the study drug or treatment is given to a large group of people (100 – 300) to see if it is effective, and to further evaluate its safety.

In phase III studies the study drug or treatment is given to a larger group of people (1,000 – 3,000) to confirm its effectiveness, monitor side effects, compare it to commonly used treatments, and collect information that will allow the drug or treatment to be used safely.

Phase – IV studies are done after the drug or treatment has been marketed. These studies continue testing the study drug or treatment to collect information about their effect in various populations and any side effects associated with long – term use.

All clinical trials are based on a set of rules called a protocol. A protocol describes what types of people may participate in the trial; the schedule of tests, procedures, medications, and dosages; and the length of the study. While in a clinical trial, participants are seen regularly by the research staff to monitor their health and to determine the safety and effectiveness of their treatment.

The major difference between a clinical trial and a prospective study is the randomized nature of the clinical trial.

The experimental and control groups must be comparable in all factors except the one being studied i.e., the drug.

One can achieve comparability on factors that are known to have an influence on the outcome, such as age, sex, race, or severity of the disease, by matching for these factors. But one cannot match individuals for factors whose influence is not known or cannot be measured.

This problem can be resolved by the random allocation of individuals to the experimental and control groups, which assures the comparability of these groups with respect to all factors – known and unknown, measurable and not measurable – except the one being studied.

Randomization is the means by which the investigator avoids introducing bias into the process of allocating individuals to the experimental or study groups.

Types of blinding

Single blinding: When the person receiving treatment or intervention (subject) is unaware of the treatment group.

Double blinding: When the subject and person noting the outcome measure (researcher) are unaware of the treatment group.

Triple blinding. When the subject, researcher and person doing analysis (statistician) are unaware of the treatment group.

Classification of clinical trial falls into big groups:

I. **Controlled trials**

    1. Parallel or concurrent controls

        a. *Randomized*

        b. *Not randomized*

    2. Sequential controls

        a. *Self-control*

        b. *Crossover*

    3. External controls

II. **Studies with no controls**

Controlled trials are studies in which the experimental drug or procedure is compared with another drug or procedure as usually previously accepted or placebo treatment.

Uncontrolled trials are studies in which the experimental drug or procedure is described being not compared with another treatment.

Because the purpose of an experiment is to determine if the intervention makes a difference, studies with controls have greater validity in medicine than uncontrolled studies.

1. **Controlled trials with concurrent (parallel) controls**

2. A **parallel study** is a type of clinical **study** where two groups of treatments, A and B, are given so that one group receives only A while another group receives only B. Other names for this type

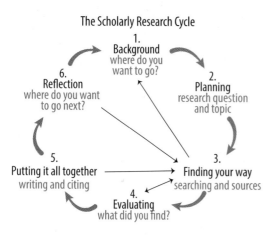

The Scholarly Research Cycle

Fig.3.6   Basis of research

of **study** include "between patient" and "non-crossover".

The more common way to make a controlled trial is to have two groups of subjects: one group receives the experimental procedure (the experimental group) and the other receives the standard procedure or placebo (the control group): The experimental and control groups, as far as possible, should be similar so that any differences between the groups will be due to the planed intervention only. It is important to provide a concurrent control: interventions for both groups are planed for the same time period and the same study.

In order to reduce the human factor, the researcher can design a **blind trial,** which means a clinical trial when the subjects do not know what intervention they are receiving. A **double-blind trial is one** in which neither the subjects nor the investigators know if the subjects are in the experimental or the control group.

Due to ethics, in clinical trials only beneficial interventions are permitted.

a   **Randomized controlled trials** provide the strongest evidence for concluding causation; they provide the best insurance

that the result was due to the intervention only.

b   In a randomized controlled trial an intervention is administered to a group that has been **randomly selected;** hence, we do not know what it is receiving (blind). Randomization provides that each individual entered in the trial has the same chance of receiving each of the possible interventions, so allocation of subjects in an experimental or a control group is given by chance. Also, randomization ensures that known and unknown confounding factors are equal in both groups. This is a way to reduce bias.

c   **Non randomized controlled trials** are studies that do not use randomized assignments. They are called clinical trials or comparative studies with no mention of randomization as well. Studies using nonrandomized controls are considered much weaker because they do nothing to prevent bias in patient assignment.

3.   **Sequential controlled trials**

a.   **Self-control trials** are studies in which the same group works as the control group. A moderate level of control can be obtained by using the same group of subjects for both experimental and control options.

b.   **Crossover trial**

The crossover study design is a repeated measures design in experimental studies where each patient is randomly assigned to a sequence of treatments, including at least two treatments (of which one "treatment" may be a standard treatment or a placebo).

There are two important issues with crossover study designs.

1.   The order effect. The order in which treatments are administered may affect the outcome. An example might be a drug with many adverse events given first; making patients taking a second, less

harmful medicine, more sensitive to any adverse effects.

2. The carry-over effect between treatments. In practice carry-over can be dealt with by use of a wash-out period between treatments, or by making observations sufficiently later after the start of a treatment period that any carry-over effect is minimized.

(1) To experimental group and another (2) in a control group. After a time, interventions are suspended and left a space (wash out period) without it. Then the intervention (1) is administered to the control group and intervention (2) is administered to the experimental group. **Trials with External Controls** are the studies when investigators compare the results of another researcher or with the results of a previous study. Also, they are called historical controls. *Analysis* of clinical trial study includes the calculation of the association measure as:

Experimental event rate (EER)

Control event rate (CER)

Relative risk (RR)

Absolute risk reduction (ARR)

Relative risk reduction (RRR)

Number needed to treat (NNT)

It is easy to calculate the association measures for a clinical trial study when the results are arranged in the 2x2 table: *1. Experimental event rate (EER)*—rate of event (risk of disease) in a group of subjects that received experimental treatment.

EER=

3. **Control event rate (CER)**—rate of event (risk of disease) in a group subjects that received traditional treatment or placebo.

4. *Relative risk (RR)*—is ratio of the risk of disease in an exposed subjects group (received experiment treatment) to the rate of risk disease in a non-exposed subjects group (did not receive experiment treatment). Relative risk indicates how more likely exposed people have an outcome then unexposed people.

The relative risk interpretation measurement scale:

RR=1, the intervention is an indifferent factor.

RR>1, intervention is a risk factor.

RR<1, intervention is a beneficial/ protective factor.

5. *Absolute risk reduction (ARR)* provides a way to assess the reduction in risk compared with the baseline risk and indicates how many subjects avoid the event occurrence for every 100 subjects. e.g.: In the aspirin study the EER for a cardiovascular disease (CVD) was 0.14 in the aspirin group (experimental group), and the control group event rate (CER) was 0.30. In this case, ARR = 0.30 – 0.14 = 0.16.

The interpretation:

The risk of CVD is 14 subjects per 100 in the group taking aspirin, and 30 in the group-taking a placebo By it taking aspirin, every 16 subjects per 100 people avoid the occurrence of CVD or 160 per 1,000 people, etc.

6. *Number needed to treat* is an added advantage of interpreting risk data in terms of absolute risk reduction. The main meaning is to find out the number needed to treat in order to prevent one event.

For e.g. in the previous example of aspirin study, NNT = 1/0.16=6.25, the number needed to treat is 6.25. Aspirin can be given to more than six patients so that secondary prevention leads to one cardiovascular disease risk reduction. This type of information helps clinicians evaluate the relative risks and benefits of a particular treatment.

7. ***Relative risk reduction (RRR)*** is defined as amount of risk reduction relative to the baseline.

RRR=CER-EER/CER=1–RR

e.g.: In the previous aspirin study RRR=0.53 or 53%

The relative risk reduction tells us that, relative to the baseline risk of 30 CVD per 100 people, giving aspirin reduces the risk by 53%.

Advantages

1. Give strong causality evidence

2. Less bias

3. Historic controls can be used in preliminary study

Disadvantages

1. Expensive

2. Ethical issues

3. Needed Time

4. Participant compliance

Basis of meta-analysis

Because the results of any one study of an issue are seldom definitive, it is often useful to combine results from many studies. Meta-analysis, described in detail by Petitti (1994), Dickersin and Berlin (1992), and Greenland (1987), is one approach to combining results. Specifically, meta-analysis is a quantitative approach for systematically combining the results of previous research in order to arrive at conclusions about the body of research as a whole (Petitti 1994). Petitti describes four steps in undertaking a meta-analysis.

1. **Identify relevant studies.** The first step in a meta-analysis is to identify the relevant studies. Systematic, explicit criteria must be established for including studies in a meta-analysis. The establishment of explicit criteria distinguishes meta-analysis from a qualitative literature review. Identifying relevant studies usually involves searching personal reference lists, computerized sources such as Medline, lists of references in other relevant original articles and review articles, the contents of journals in which relevant articles are likely to be published, and doctoral dissertations on the topic. Experts in the area are usually consulted to determine if they know of articles that have been missed through the other sources. In addition, it is important to try to identify unpublished studies, because of "publication bias"—the greater tendency of research with statistically significant results to be submitted and published than results that are not statistically significant and/or null. In other words, published studies are generally not representative of all studies that have been undertaken of an issue. When identifying studies from these various sources, one usually starts with a very broad list of potential studies for inclusion and then narrows it down to studies that are indeed relevant. It should be apparent that identification of relevant studies is usually a time consuming process.

2. **Inclusion/Exclusion criteria.** The second step in a meta-analysis is deciding upon inclusion and exclusion criteria for the studies under consideration as relevant.

The criteria should be established before data abstraction begins. Criteria for inclusion usually specify the study designs to be included, the years of publication or of data collection, the languages in which the articles are written (e.g. English only or English plus other specified languages), which publication will be selected when more than one publication based on the same or overlapping data is available, the minimum sample size and the extent of follow-up, the treatments and/or exposures, the manner in which the exposures, treatment, and outcomes were measured, and the completeness of information. Finally, study quality needs to be considered. As a minimum, studies whose quality is so poor (by some pre-specified criteria) that the results are likely to be invalid should not be included in the meta-analysis. Rating scales may be developed to assess the quality of the included studies. On this basis, studies may be stratified into two or more groups according to their quality. Although in theory studies could be weighted by their score on the rating scale, this has not been done in practice.

3. **Data abstraction**. The third step in a meta-analysis is data abstraction. The first component of data abstraction is documenting whether or not each identified study is eligible for inclusion. Then, data on the results of the study and characteristics of the study such as its design, number of participants, and other important features are abstracted. The abstraction should produce data that are reliable, valid, and free of bias. Blinding the abstractor to aspects of the study that might influence the data abstraction is the best way to minimize bias in data abstraction.

4. **Statistical analysis and exploration of heterogeneity**. The final step in conducting a meta-analysis is statistical analysis and exploration of heterogeneity if it is present. The analysis generally involves combining the data to obtain a summary estimate of the measure of association, together with its variance and 95% confidence limits. In some situations, dose-response relationships may be presented. The reader is referred to Petitti (1994), Dickersin and Berlin (1992), and Greenland (1987), for further discussion of statistical analysis. Whether the effect is homogenous across studies should be specifically examined and tested; if not

homogenous, reasons for heterogeneity should be sought. An increasingly important use of meta-analysis is to identify reasons for discrepancies in study results.

Application of meta-analysis

Although meta-analysis is a quite popular way of summarizing data from several studies, its use has generated a fair amount of controversy, particularly when used to combine results of observational studies (Shapiro 1994 a, b; Petitti 1994; Greenland 1994). The quality of the meta-analysis depends upon rigorous adherence to the methodology described above, and especially upon delineation of the criteria for selection of the specific studies eligible for inclusion in the meta-analysis. Articles based on meta-analysis need to be read in the same critical manner as original articles. When studies arrive at different conclusions or there are large differences among studies in their estimates of effect size, meta-analysis is most appropriately used to try to identify the reasons for heterogeneity and to suggest further areas for research—not to calculate a single summary estimate of effect (Greenland 1994; Petitti 1994). When properly done, meta-analysis provides a way of summarizing literature that is less subjective than the usual qualitative review. Notwithstanding concerns about meta-analysis, it has become an extremely important tool in the formulation of public health and clinical policy, and especially in the development of guidelines. A recent example can be seen in the American College of Physicians Guidelines on the Use of Hormone Replacement Therapy, which conducted separate meta-analyses of studies of hormone replacement therapy and coronary artery disease, hip fracture, and breast and endometrial cancer to derive estimates of the relative risk of these conditions. It used this information as input to a decision model estimating life-expectancy in users and nonusers of hormone replacement therapy

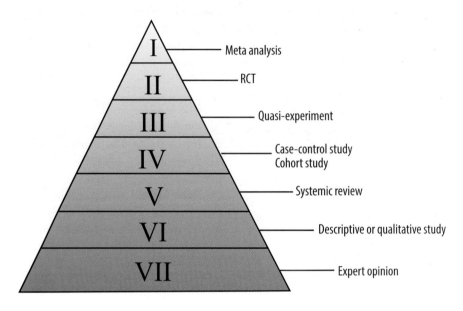

Fig.3.7 Levels of evidence

(Grady et al. 1992). It is likely that the use of meta-analysis for these purposes will increase, not diminish.

Levels of evidence (Fig.3.7):

Lev el I: Evidence from a systematic review of all relevant randomized controlled trial (RCT)

Level II: Evidence from well designed RCT

Level III: Evidence from well designed quasi experimental study

Level IV: Evidence from well designed case control and cohort study

Level V: Evidence from systematic reviews of descriptive and qualitative studies

Level VI: Evidence from a descriptive or qualitative study

Level VII: Evidence from opinions of authorities of expert committees

Guidance on interpreting epidemiologic evidence

Epidemiologic studies have contributed a great deal to the practice of public health. They provide information that is used on a day-to-day basis to select interventions and to counsel patients about risk. They are important input to clinical guidelines and a variety of policy decisions in the applied setting.

Selection of study design

In selecting the design of the study you have to consider the type of information you want to obtain and devise strategies to enable you to obtain that information.

The selection of an appropriate study design depends on:

1. The state of knowledge about the problem

2. The nature of the problem and its environment

3. The resources available for the research

4. Objectives of the research

5. The ingenuity and creativity

Chapter

4 SAMPLING

The procedure of selecting a certain number of study units from a defined population is called Sampling. A representative sample has all important characteristics of the population from which it is drawn. A representative sample is the one with which we can draw valid inference regarding the population characteristics.

Terms used in sampling

The following terms are commonly used in Sampling.

Universe

A specified group (usually very large) of the persons, objects, measurements or values

Population

A study group of the persons and objects in which specific measurements or values are obtained

- Study population
- Target population
- Reference population

Study Unit

Every unit included in the study is called a Study Unit. The study unit can be a:

- Person
- Household
- Family
- School
- Patient with a particular disease
- Patient undergoing a particular surgical procedure
- Patient receiving a particular medicine

Study subjects

A full description of the subjects (sample) or participants involved in the research. The demographic information, socio economical characteristics or health profile may be required.

- Describe sampling of the study population
- Define the number of participants
- Participant criteria
- Describe sample selection (age, gender, ethnicity, income bracket, etc.), characteristics related to the disease of interest, etc.

Sample selection

How will the participants be selected? The criteria for becoming a participant are determined as follows:

1. Inclusion criteria
2. Exclusion criteria

Sampling frame

It is the listing of all units of the population from which the sample is to be drawn.

An important issue influencing the choice of the most appropriate sample is whether a sampling frame is available or not.

Advantages of sampling

- By drawing a sample from a larger population, cost of the study is reduced considerably.
- The study can be done with greater speed i.e., in less time.
- And with greater accuracy.
- Drawing a sample can increase the scope of a study since several aspects can be studied.
- Some tests which are not possible in the population can be applied to a smaller population and important information can be obtained.
- Study can be in depth and more subtle.
- Study of the entire universe is unnecessary and not cost-effective.

Fundamentals of Sampling

Since sampling is expected to represent the whole population, the sampling procedure is to follow three fundamentals:

1. It has to be representative of the reference population so that the results from the sample can be generalized.
2. The sample is sufficiently large. The sample size is scientifically calculated.
3. The selected units have been properly approached, included and interviewed/examined.

The way a sample is drawn is one of the most crucial aspects of research.

Types of sampling

There are two major types of sampling procedures:

- Probability sampling.
- Non probability sampling.

Probability sampling

When each sampling unit has an equal and known chance of being included in the sample.

Non probability sampling

When sampling units do not have an equal chance of being included in the sample.

Probability sampling

Probability sampling involves selecting procedures to ensure that all study units have an equal and/or known chance of being included in the study.

- Simple random sampling
- Systematic random sampling
- Stratified sampling
- Cluster sampling
- Multi-stage sampling

Simple random sampling

In simple random sample, every sampling unit in the sampling frame has the same chance of being selected (Table 4.1).

For selecting a simple random sample:

1. We need to make a numbered list of all the study units in the population from which we want to draw a sample. This is called the Sampling Frame.
2. Then we can select the required number of sampling units using a lottery method or random number tables or a computer programme like SPSS, Epi-Calc.

Table 4.1   Simple random sampling

Advantages	Disadvantages
• Because every unit in the population has an equal chance of being included in the sample, the sample is assured of being representative and subject only to sampling error.	• If the sampling frame is large, this method may be impracticable because of the difficulty and expense of constructing or updating it in large-scale surveys.
• Estimates are easy to calculate.	• Minority subgroups of interest in the population may not be present in the sample in sufficient numbers for study.

Table 4.2   Systemic random sampling

Advantages	Disadvantages
• The sample is easy to select.	• The sample may be biased if a hidden periodicity in the population coincides with that of the selection.
• A suitable sampling frame can be identified more easily.	• It is difficult to assess the precision of the estimate from one survey.
• The sample is evenly spread over the entire reference population.	

Table 4.3   Stratified sampling

Advantages	Disadvantages
• Every unit in a stratum has the same chance of being selected.	• The sampling frame of the entire population has to be prepared separately for each stratum.
• Using the same sampling fraction for all strata ensures proportionate representation in the sample of the characteristics being studied.	• Varying the sampling fraction between strata, to ensures selection of sufficient numbers in minority subgroups for study, affects the proportional representativeness of the subgroups in the sample as a whole.
• Adequate representation of minority groups of interest can be ensured by stratification and by varying the sampling fraction between strata as required.	

Systematic random sampling

In systematic random sampling, the sampling units are selected at regular intervals (e.g. every 5th, 15th, 34th) from the sampling frame.

Ideally, we randomly select a number to tell us where to start selecting individuals from the list (Table 4.2).

Stratified sampling

If it is important that the sample includes the representative groups of study units with specific characteristics e.g. residents from urban and rural areas of different age groups, then the sampling frame must be divided into groups or STRATA according to these characteristics. A simple random sample of predetermined size will then be obtained from each group (stratum) (Table 4.3).

Cluster sampling

This is often a convenient method, especially when there is no sampling frame showing all individual subjects.

- The population is first divided into clusters of homogeneous units, usually based on geographical contiguity like (villages) or organizational units (clinics, factories, schools).

- A sample of such clusters is then selected. All the units in the selected clusters are studied.

Multi-stage sampling

In very large and diverse populations, sampling may be done in two or more stages.

This is often the case in community based studies, where the people are to be contacted in different villages and villages are to be chosen from different areas.

Selection is done in stages until the final sampling units (for example, households or persons) are arrived at.

- In the first stage, a list of large-sized sampling units is prepared. These may be towns, or villages or schools.

- A sample of these is selected at random, with probability of selection proportional to size.

- For each of the selected first-stage units, a list of smaller sampling units is prepared. (For example, if the first-stage units are towns, then the second-stage units may be houses or households).

- A sample of these second-stage units is then randomly selected from each of the selected first-stage units. These are then studied.

The sampling procedure is carried out in phases as shown in the following example.

A study of health care utilization is to be carried out in a district and 150 households are to be interviewed. The district has six tehsils and

Table 4.4   Convenience sampling

Advantages	Disadvantages
• Cuts down on the cost of preparing a sampling frame	• Sampling error is usually higher than for a simple random sample of the same size.
• Cuts down on the cost of travelling between selected units	
• Eliminates the problem of packing (in health surveys), especially those involving case finding and treatment	

Table 4.5   Purposive Sampling

Advantages	Disadvantages
It cuts down the cost of preparing a sampling frame.	Sampling error is increased compared with a simple random sample of the same size.

each tehsil has 10 to 15 villages. The sample will be selected as under:

- Select three tehsils out of six, by simple random sampling.
- From each tehsil, select five villages by simple random sampling.
- From each village, select 10 households by systematic random sampling.

Non-probability sampling

When there is no assurance that each element will have the same chance of being included in the sample

There are following major types:

1. Convenience sampling
2. Purposive sampling
3. Quota sampling
4. Snow-ball sampling
5. Temporal sampling

Convenience sampling

In this method, the study units that happen to be available at the time of data collection are selected in the sample. For example, you may select the first 10 patients reporting to a clinic or all students present in the library at a particular time.

The sample selected in such a manner is unlikely to be representative. The purpose for such sampling is usually exploratory e.g. to get the feel of the situation (Table 4.4).

Purposive sampling

This method consists of selecting study units on the basis of some pre-determined idea e.g. clinical knowle.g. or those with a particular characteristic. For example, samples from different age groups or all those suffering from a particular disease e.g. all hypertensives.

The results of such a sample cannot be generalized (Table 4.5).

Quota sampling

In this type of sampling, the segments of the population are identified and the researcher determines the proportions of elements needed from the various segments.

This method ensures that a certain number of study units from different categories with specific characteristics appear in the sample so that all these characteristics are represented.

For example, if a study is to be conducted to know the opinion of various types of people about the utility of a health institution in a locality, then a simple random sample may not include key informants like political, religious, or educational leaders. So the researcher may decide to include a certain number of each category to be interviewed.

Snowball sampling

In this method, the individuals with certain characteristics are asked to identify similar individuals for inclusion in the study.

Temporal sampling

This method entails including all cases occurring in a specified period of time e.g. all

Table 4.6   Advantages/Disadvantages of Probability and Non-probability Sampling

Advantages	Disadvantages
Probability Sampling	Expensive
Minimum bias	Inconvenient
Allows estimation of sampling error	Problematic with large populations
More authentic	Technically skilled operator needed
Non-probability sample	
Convenient	Results cannot be generalized
Economical	Maximum bias
Less time consuming	Authenticity debatable
Less skilled operator required	Weaker type of sampling

patients of myocardial infarction reporting to a CCU during one week.

Sampling procedure

An important issue influencing the choice of the most appropriate sample is whether a sampling frame is available or not. A sampling frame is the listing of all the units that form the study population.

If a sampling frame is not available, it is not possible to sample the study units in such a way that the probability for the different units to be selected in the sample is known. In such cases, use **Non Probability Sampling.**

If the sampling frame exists or can be compiled, each study unit has the sample. Therefore, **Probability Sampling** should be used (Table 4.6).

Chapter 5

DATA COLLECTION AND PRESENTATION

Data collection and presentation techniques allow the researcher to systematically collect information about subjects of study (people, objects, phenomena) and about the settings in which they occur. In the collection of data, researchers have to be systematic. If data are collected haphazardly, it will be difficult to answer research questions in a conclusive way.

Data collection tools

Tools should be valid and reliable:

Considered valid if they measure what they purport to measure.

Reliability refers to the consistency and reproducibility of the results.

- Internal consistency is the degree to which all items in a domain reflect the same construct.

- In the classical model of validity, construct validity is one of three main types of validity evidence, along side content validity and criterion validity. Three types of validity are content, criterion and construct validity. Pilot studies are commonly used to check the validity of the data collection tool.

Data collection procedures

a **Observing behaviours and attitudes of participants:** This method specifies the conditions and methods at making observation. In this method, the information is sought by way of the investigator's own direct observation without asking from the respondent. The main advantage of this method is that subjective bias is eliminated, if observations are done accurately. It most commonly uses the check lists or proformas.

b **Questionnaire method:** Under this method, a list of questions pertaining to the survey (known as a questionnaire) is prepared and sent to the various informants by post. The questionnaire contains questions and provides space for answers. A request is made to the informants through a covering letter to fill up the questionnaire and send it back within a specified time. The respondents have to answer the questions on their own. The questionnaire can be delivered directly hand by hand, through surface post or as an electronic questionnaire.

In preparing a research questionnaire general question, question wording to collect personal information, use of unfamiliar terms and jargon, etc. should be avoided. Further, before distribution of a research ·questionnaire at least two pre-tests should be conducted. A written questionnaire (also referred to as a self-administered questvionnaire) is a data collection tool in which written questions are presented that are to be answered by the respondents in written form. A written questionnaire can be

Table 5.1   Use of open and closed questions

	Use Open	Use Closed
Purpose	Actual words or quotes	Most common answers
Respondents	Capable to provide answers	Willing to answer only if easy and quick
Asking the questions	Choice are unknown	Choice can be anticipated
Analyzing results	Content analyses; time consuming	Counting or scoring
Reporting results	Individual or grouped responses	Statistical data

Source: Beth Dawson, Robert G. Trapp, Basic and Clinical Biostatistics 2004

administered in different ways, such as by sending questionnaires by mail with clear instructions on how to answer the questions and asking for mailed responses. Gathering all or part of the respondents in one place at one time, giving oral or written instructions, and letting the respondents fill out the questionnaires; or hand-delivering questionnaires to respondents and collecting them later.

Questionnaires with fixed or closed questions are on topics about which little is known. Open-ended questions without guidelines on how to ask (or to answer) them; comprehensive phrased questions; 'leading questions' that cause the respondent to believe one answer would be preferred over another; or questions placed in an illogical order. Weighing scales or other measuring equipment that are not standardized. These sources of bias can be prevented by carefully planning the data collection process and by pre-testing the data collection tools.

c   **Interview Method:** This involves listening to or integrating informants. The interview method of collecting data involves presentation of oral-verbal stimuli

and reply in terms of oral – verbal responses. So, under this method of collecting data, there is a face to face contact with the persons from whom the information is to be collected. The interviewer asks them questions pertaining to the survey and collects the desired information. This method can be used through personal interview, telephone interview, chat, audio conferencing, video conferencing, etc. The interview can be structured, semi-structured or an open interview.

d   **Schedules method:** In this method of data collection, the enumerator or interviewers who are specially appointed for the purpose along with schedules, go to the respondents, put to them the questions from the performa in the order the questionnaire is listed and record the replies in the space meant for the same in the performa. In certain situations, schedules may be handed over to respondents and enumerators may help them in recording their answer to various questions in the said schedules. The enumerator explains the aims and objectives of the investigation and also removes the difficulties which respondents may feel in relation to understanding the implication of a particular question, or a definition or concept of a difficult term. This method has the advantage over the questionnaire method in the sense that the respondents have no scope to misunderstand any question and thereby giving an irrelevant answer.

e **Information from correspondents:** Under this method, the investigator appoints local agents or correspondents in different places to collect information. These correspondents collect and transmit information to the central office where the data are processed. The special advantage of this method is that it is cheap and appropriate for extensive investigation. However, it may not always ensure accurate results because of the personal prejudice and bias of the correspondents. Newspaper agencies generally adopt this method.

f **Focus group discussions**

A focus group discussion allows a group of 8–12 informants to freely discuss a certain subject with the guidance of a facilitator or reporter. Focus research and develop relevant research hypotheses.

Exploring in greater depth the problem to be investigated. Formulate appropriate questions for more structured, larger scale surveys. Help understand and solve unexpected problems in interventions. Develop appropriate messages for health education programmes and later evaluate the messages for clarity. Explore controversial topics with ethical considerations.

Besides the above methods, nowadays many big companies also follow some other method for primary data collection like distributor or store audit, clients or patients panels, projective techniques, depth interviews, content analysis, etc.

The secondary data can be collected by way of examining historical and other records, literature and proverbs. If data available in secondary sources are reliable, suitable and adequate then only the secondary data should be collected.

Presentation of data

Table 5.2   Use of open and closed questions

	Self administered by mail/email	Self administered, in person	Interview by phone	Interview in person
Cost	+ +	+	-	-
Time	+ +	+	-	-
Standardization	+	+	+/-	+/-
Depth/details	-	-	+	+ +
Response rate	-	+ +	+	+ +
Missing Response	-	+	+ +	+ +

+Advantages; - Disadvantage; +/-Neutral

Source: Beth Dawson, Robert G. Trapp, Basic and Clinical Biostatistics, 2004

Table 5.3   One way table

Gender of the patient				
Valid	Frequancy	Percentage	Valid percentage	Cumulative percentage
Male	3053	59.5	59.5	59.5
Female	2074	40.5	40.5	100.0
Total	5127	100.0	100.0	

Table 5.4   One way table

Respondent's sex Race of respondent crosstabulation				
Count Respondent's sex	Race of respondent crosstabulation			Total
	White	Black	Other	
Male	545	71	20	636
Female	719	133	29	881
Total	1264	204	49	1517

Tables

The table is commonly used for data presentation and has the following components.

Title

A title is a heading at the top of the table. The title should be brief and self explanatory.

Column captions and box-head

The headings for different columns are called column captions and this part of the column caption is called the box-head. The column caption should be in brief, clear and arranged in order of importance.

Row caption and stub

The headings for different rows are called row captions and the part of the table containing row captions is called the stub. The row captions should be brief, clear and arranged in order of importance.

The tables are commonly used to display data observation:

a. Simple Frequency Distribution Table (S.F.D.T.)

Table: Distribution of students at the University of Medicine of Moldova according to their gender

Graphs

Graphs just represent a summary of data that has been collected to support a particular theory. It is usually suggested that the graphic representation of the data should be looked at before proceeding for format statistical analysis.

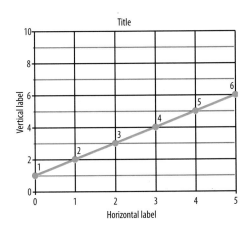

Fig.5.1   Line diagram

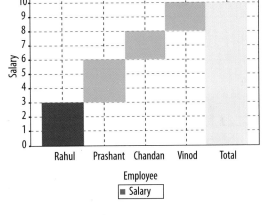

Fig.5.4   Bar graph

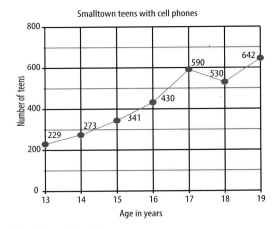

Fig.5.2   Line diagram

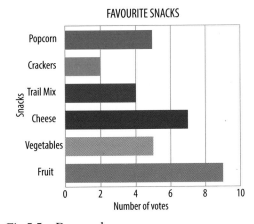

Fig.5.5   Bar graph

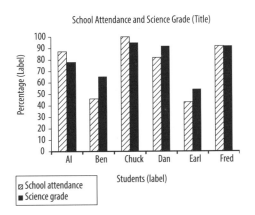

Fig.5.3   Bar graphs

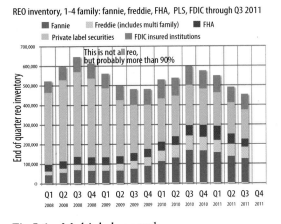

Fig.5.6   Multiple bar graph

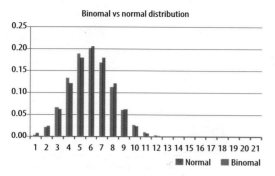

Fig.5.7   Bar graphs

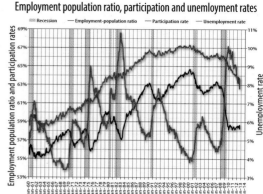

Fig.5.10   Comparison of three data sets

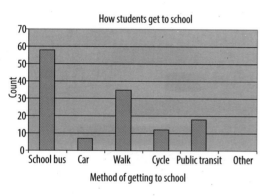

Fig.5.8   Bar graph

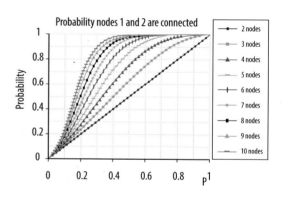

Fig.5.11   Probability graphs

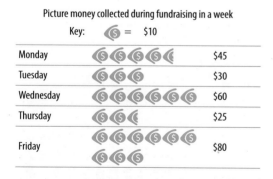

Fig.5.9   Picture graph

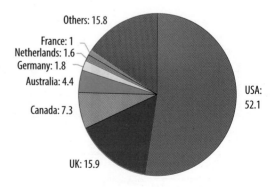

Fig.5.12   Pie diagram

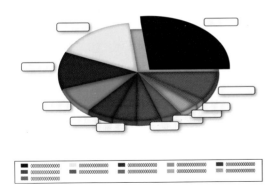

Fig.5.13   Pie diagram

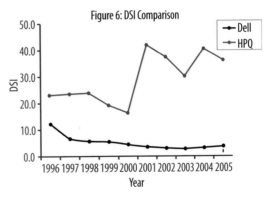

Fig.5.15   Comparison of two data sets

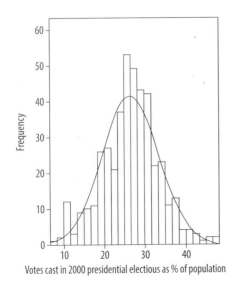

Fig.5.14   Histogram

Common uses of graphs

- Visual representation (good to understand and attractive)
- To check assumptions
- Help in selection of statistical tools

Types of graph

- Line graph
- Simple bar diagram

- Multiple bar diagram
- Subdivided bar diagram
- Pie diagram
- Histogram
- Scatter plots
- Box Plot
- Line graphs
- Bar graphs
- Picture graphs
- Point graphs
- Probability graphs
- Pie diagrams

Histograms

The most informative way to present relative frequencies. A histogram looks a bit like a column chart, but:

Whereas a column chart is a pictorial representation of a frequency distribution of either nominal or ordinal data *(categorical data)*, a histogram display a frequency distribution for discrete or continuous data *(numerical data)*.

Histograms give an idea of the shape of the relative frequency distribution. Column charts are just tallies and can't tell about distribution shapes.

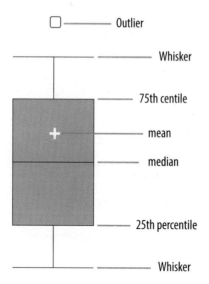

Fig.5.16   Box plots

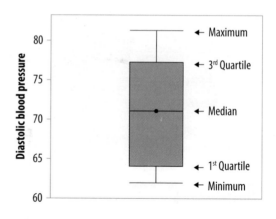

Fig.5.18   Box plots

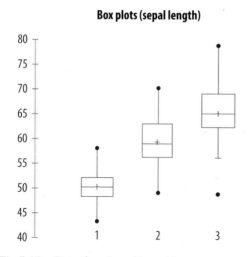

Fig.5.17   Box plots (sepal length)

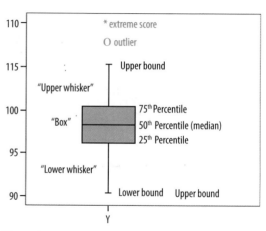

Fig.5.19   Box plots

- The horizontal axis displays the true limits of the various intervals. The vertical axis displays the absolute or relative frequencies values.

Frequency polygons

Another commonly used graph, it is similar to the histogram in many aspects. A frequency polygon uses the same two axes as a histogram. It is constructed by placing a point at the center of each interval such that the height of the point is equal to the absolute or relative frequency associated with the interval. Points are also placed on the horizontal axis at the midpoints of the intervals immediately preceding and immediately following the intervals that contain observations. Straight lines then connect the points. As in a histogram the frequency of observations for particular intervals is represented by the area within the interval beneath the line segment. The

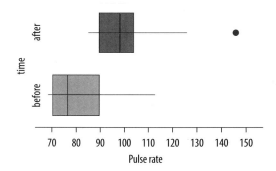

Fig.5.20   Box plots

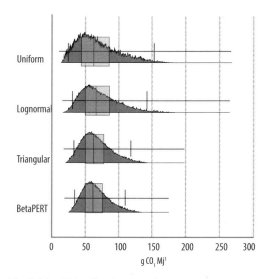

Fig.5.21   Distribution graphs

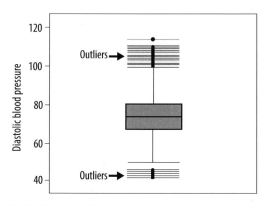

Fig.5.22   Box plots—outliers

frequency polygons are superior to histograms because they can easily be superimposed for comparing two or more sets of data.

Box plots

It is used to summarize a set of discrete or continuous observations when there is more then one group. That way of presentation shows only the summary of the data and no information about every point in the group. The central box, that can be depicted vertically or horizontally, extends from 25th to 75th percentiles of the data set. The line running between marks the 50th percentiles of the data set. If this line lies approximately halfway between the two quartiles, it means that the data set distribution is roughly symmetric.

The lines projecting out to the box represent the adjacent values of the plot which are the

Table 5.5   Relation of graph with data type

Graph type	Data type
Pie chart	Qualitative data (ideally with less categories)
Bar chart	Qualitative data (ideally when more categories), discreet data
Multiple or sub divided bar charts	Qualitative data with multi way
Histogram	For quantitative data (especially for continuous)
Scatter diagram	To see the relationship of two quantitative data
Box plot	To see the outlier in quantitative data

most extreme observations, but not more than 1.5 times interquartile range. All points outside this range are represented by circles. These observations are considered to be outliers or data points that are not typical of the rest of the values.

Nominal and ordinal data presentation

Nominal and ordinal data presentations are as follows:

1. Relative values: The types and methods of calculation. Graph presentation

2. Vital statistics indicators. Tables and graph presentation

3. Adjusted rate: Direct method of standardization. Tables and graph presentation

Relative values

As usually obtained statistic information in a research is presented by *absolute values.* These values are difficult to interpret because they are not able to make a comparison, synthesis or correlation among different characteristics.

To make comparisons among groups more meaningful, relative values may be used instead of absolute numbers.

Relative value types

- Rate
- Proportion
- Ratio

Rates are intensive statistical indicators expressing the frequency (the level) of a phenomenon computed over a specified period of time.

Rate=

a – number of observations with a given characteristic (such as those who died in a specified year and place)

$a+b$ – total number of observation (such as number of population)

base – is a multiplier (e.g. 100 (%); 1,000 (0/00); 10,000 (0/000); 100,000 (0/0000)

Rates are mostly used to establish the morbidity, natality and mortality phenomenon and allow:

- To determine the frequency of a phenomenon spreading in a specified research group

- To make a comparison of different groups by their frequency level of a homogenous phenomenon

- To detect the dynamic changes in the phenomenon frequency spreading on the base of a specified research group

Graph presentation: Line graph, bar chart, column chart

Proportions are extensive statistical indicators expressing the structure of a phenomenon. A proportion is defined as a part of a phenomenon divided by the whole phenomenon. Mostly this indicator is shown in %.

Proportion (percentage) =

The proportion is a static indicator, which never makes the association between medium and phenomenon and never allows the evaluation of its dynamic changes: it makes balance statistics in a specified moment of time only.

Graph presentation: Pie chart

Ratios are the rapport between two independent phenomenons. It is defined as a part divided by another part. So, the ratio is the number of observations in a group with a given characteristic divided by the number of observations without the given characteristic:

Ratio =

Graph presentation: line graph, bar chart, column chart

Vital statistics indicators

Vital statistics describe the life of the population: births, deaths, marriages, divorces, and diseases occurrences.

Mostly vital statistical indicators are represented by rates. Some of the most commonly used rates are briefly defined in the following items:

Mortality rate

The number of deaths that occur during the specified time period, divided by the total number of population who were at the risk of dying for the same period of time.

A crude rate is a rate computed over all individuals in a given entire population, regardless of differences caused by age, gender, race, etc. Rates that are computed within relatively small, well-defined subgroups are called *specific rates.*

Mortality rate calculated for individual age groups are known as *age-specific death rates;* for individual sex groups – *sex-specific mortality rate;* for cause groups – *cause-specific mortality rate.*

Morbidity rate

The number of persons who develop a disease during the specified time period divided by the number of people who were at risk for the same period of time.

Incidence and prevalence are the main measures of morbidity and are commonly used to evaluate the population health status in many medical and epidemiological researches.

Incidence is defined as the number of new cases that have occurred during the specified time period divided by the number of people who were at risk for the same period of time.

Prevalence is defined as the number of persons with a given disease at a given point in time divided by the population at risk for that disease at that time.

Prevalence and Incidence rates are used to evaluate disease patterns and make future projections.

The morbidity rate provides a standard way to evaluate the crude rate and the specific rate as well.

Example:

In a specified year and locality the number of population is 75,000. In that year were born 1908 and died 897 of individuals. In that locality were 40 doctors: 20 – physicians; 10 – surgeons; 10 – other.

Compute all main possible statistical indicators.

1. *Rates: (intensive indicators)*

    Birth rate=0/00

    Crude mortality rate=0/00

2. *Proportion (extensive indicator)*

    Percentage of physicians=Percentage of surgeons—the same way that is considered up.

3. *Ratio (rapport indicator)*

    Medical supply = 5.3 doctors for every 10,000 populations

Adjusted rate: Direct method of standardization

Crude rates can be used to make comparisons between two different populations only if the populations are homogenous in all characteristics. Therefore if the populations are different by factors such as gender, age, etc., instead of a crude rate, an adjusted crude rate by gender, age, etc., must be used for comparison otherwise the comparison will not be valid.

The direct method of standardization focuses on computing the conventional rates that would result if instead of having different characteristics distribution, all groups being compared were to have the same standard composition. So, adjusted rates are conventional values (not real) that make sense only for the comparison process and cannot to be used separately.

Determining an adjusted rate is a relatively simple process having the following steps:

1. To compute the rates for each comparison group

2. To select the standard distribution

3. To compute the expected number for each group

4. To calculate the adjusted rate for each group

Types of data collection

Data collection is performed in a research process for:

1. Data for quality management of research

The data collection for quality management of research is very important and includes:

- Protocol review and approval
- Documentation of standard operating procedures (SOPs)
- Validation of research instruments
- Training the project team
- Quality control and monitoring
- Evaluation of services provided
- Evaluation of the performance of service providers
- Review of reports

2. Data for research planning

Resources, including staff, equipment, supplies, logistics support, and funds

- Adherence to the research design procedures

- The research team's communication and co-ordination with the study population and other collaborating groups
- Steps researchers will take to assess the progress of the project and identify who will use the evaluation findings
- Describes information needed, sources and evaluation methods and instruments
- Examines how the project objectives will be met
- Tracks the expected impact of the intervention
- Demonstrates that the scope of the evaluation is appropriate

Methods of data collection for monitoring and evaluation

The data is collected by the following methods for monitoring, evaluation, and planning.

1. Information log and checklists

2. A formal survey and questionnaires

3. A series of key informant interviews

The vigorous data collection and presentation helped in achieving research data analysis and statistical procedures for interpretation and drawing sound conclusions for good research practices.

Chapter 6

BIOSTATISTICS AND DATA ANALYSIS

BIOSTATISTICS DEFINITIONS

BIOSTATISTICS

The word statistics is a Latin word derived from *status* meaning information useful to the state, e.g. the sizes of the populations and armed forces.

It is defined as the procedures and techniques used to collect, process and analyze data to make inferences and to reach decisions in the face of uncertainty.

Statistics refers to numerical facts obtained from the sample populations.

Field of statistics—how data are:

* presented,
* calculated,
* analysed, and
* interpreted.
* When the data we use are biological, medical or health related, the subject is called **Biostatistics.**

Basic biostatistics

Population

A collection of individuals who share a common trait

Sample

A selection of individuals from a population or set of possible observations

Types:

* Random—all are equally likely to be selected.
* Systematic—an algorithm is used to randomly select a subset.
* Stratified—there is separate representation of more than one subgroup.
* Cluster—these are grouped in space/time to reduce costs.
* Convenience—non-random sampling.

Data

Information collected about a sample or population.

Facts and figures are collected, summarised and analysed.

There are three classes of data listed with examples:

* **Discrete:** number of strokes experienced
* **Continuous:** serum cholesterol, hemoglobin, age
* **Categorical:** gender, marital status. These are further divided into two types:
  1. Nominal. When different categories cannot be ordered in any specific sequence. e.g. males, females
  2. Ordinal. When different categories can be ordered in any specific sequence e.g. fair, good, excellent

Element: An entity on which measurements are obtained

Observation: Set of measurements obtained for each element

Mean

Sum of all values (Σ) divided by number of observations. It is denoted by x.

- Advantages
  - o Easy to calculate
  - o Gives an idea of central tendency
- Disadvantages
  - o Influenced by extreme values
  - o May not convey proper sense e.g. mean number of children may turn out to be 5.77

Median

When the data is arranged in ascending or descending order, the median is the value that divides the data into two equal parts.

- Advantages

  Not influenced by extreme values
- Disadvantages
  - o Not very precise measure
  - o Not amenable to further statistical evaluation

Calculation of median

3. Arrange all values in ascending or descending order.
4. Add an to the number of observations.
5. Divide by two.
6. The answer will be the number of observations, which constitutes the median.

Mode

The figure that is occurring most in the data set is called the mode e.g. In 1, 2, 3, 4, 4, 5, 6, 7, 8, 9, the mode is 4. A mode is usually used in medicine to present bimodal distribution. Bimodal distribution means two peaks in a data set. For example, the measurements of temperature in a patient of dengue fever show bimodal distribution.

Standard deviation

- It is a measure, which describes how much individual measures differ, on average, from the mean.
- It is denoted by d or SD.
- It is the most important measure of dispersion around the mean and forms the basis of most statistical analysis.

Calculation of standard deviation

- Add all observations.
- Calculate mean.
- Find the deviation of each observation from the mean.
- Square each deviation and add them.
- Divide this sum by number of observations–1(n-1). This is called a degree of freedom.
- Take square root.

Use of Standard deviation in data set

- **Mean ± 1 SD = 68.2 % 68 %**
- **Mean ± 2 SD = 95.4 % 95 %**
- **Mean ± 3 SD = 99.7 % 99 %**

Normal distribution

Most common distribution in health related data set.

The main features:

1. **Symmetrical about its mean**
2. **Bell shaped**
3. **Mean, median and mode lie at same point**

4. Majority of continuous variables have this distribution

5. Based on the **central limit theorem** which states that if a random sample is taken from a normal distribution, the sample mean will be an estimate of the population mean

6. Parametric tests based on normal distribution of data

7. Normal distribution can be summarized by its mean and standard deviation

Skewed distribution

It is asymmetrical distribution and mean, median, and mode lie at different points. It has following types.

1. Positive skewed distribution

2. Negative skewed distribution

Non parametric tests are applied when the data show skewed distribution.

Probability

It is a measure of chance or uncertainty. It is the chance of rejecting a true null hypothesis.

Statistical significance

- The probability that the statistical association found between the variables is due to random chance

- The preset probability is set sufficiently low that one would act on the result; frequently p = 0.05

- When statistical tests result in a probability less than the preset limit, the results are said to be statistically significant, i.e. p<0.05

Clinical significance

- A measure of clinical usefulness, e.g. 1 mmHg BP reduction may be statistically significant, but may not be clinically significant

- Depends on factors such as cost, availability, patient compliance and side effects; in addition to statistical significance

Pre-test probability

An estimate of the likelihood a particular patient has a given disease based on known factors

Post-test probability

- Revision of the probability of disease after a patient has been interviewed and examined. The calculation process can be more explicit using results from epidemiologic studies, knowledge of the accuracy of tests and Bayes' theorem.

- The post-test probability from the clinical examination is the basis of consideration when ordering diagnostic tests or imaging studies. After each investigation the resultant post-test probability becomes the pre-test probability when considering new investigations.

Intention-to-treat

A strategy for analyzing data in which all participants are included in the group to which they were assigned, whether or not they completed the requirements of that group. This is to limit the bias introduced by issues of compliance.

Relative risk (RR)

Ratio of the incidence of a health outcome among the exposed population to the incidence of the health outcome in the non-exposed population.

Attributable risk

- Rate of a health outcome attributable to a hypothetical risk factor for that outcome

- [incidence in exposed population]—[incidence in non-exposed]
- Attributable risk assumes causation

Odds ratio (OR)

- Ratio of the odds of exposure to a hypothetical risk factor among cases to the odds of exposure among non-cases.
- Can be interpreted as the ratio of odds of developing the outcome (i.e. disease) among those exposed to the hypothetical risk factor to those who are not exposed.
- Odds ratio approximates Relative Risk when the prevalence of disease in the population is low.

Statistical hypothesis

- Null (Ho) no relationship exists between the two stated variables, i.e. no association between the proposed risk factor and the disease.
- Alternative (H_1) relationship does exist between the two stated variables.

Type I error (alpha error)

The null hypothesis is falsely rejected, i.e. declaring an effect to be present when it is not; the probability of this error is denoted by the p value.

Type II error (beta error)

The null hypothesis is falsely accepted, i.e. declaring a difference/effect to be absent when it is present can also be used to calculate statistical power.

Confidence interval (CI)

It provides a range of values within which the true population mean lies frequently reported as 95% CI, i.e. one can be 95% certain that the true value is within this data range.

Accuracy

How closely a measurement approaches the true value

Reliability

How consistent a measurement is when performed by different observers under the same conditions, or the same observer under different conditions. Repeated measures should produce the same results.

Measurement error

Refers to the closeness with which the measurement approaches the true value, and reliability or reproducibility refers to the extent to which the same measurement is obtained on the same occasion by the same observer, on multiple occasions by the same observer, or by different observers on the same occasion. Precision refers to the amount of variation around the measurement or estimate; a precise measure will have a small amount of variation around it.

Measurement error is said to be **differential** when the magnitude of the error for one variable differs according to the actual value of another variable. Differential measurement error can cause associations to be overestimated or underestimated, depending on the circumstances.

Measurement error is said to be **non-differential** when the magnitude of the error in one variable does not vary according to the actual value of the other variable of interest. In a 2 x 2 table, non-differential misclassification always causes the relative risk or odds ratio to be closer to 1.0, provided that errors in measurement of the two variables are independent of each other.

Validity

- Extent to which a measurement approaches what it is designed to measure.

- Determined by the accuracy of a test and comparison with control. The validity is further divided into:
  1. Internal validity
  2. External validity

Confounding

- Occurs when a variable (confounder) is related to both the exposure and outcome but is not measured, or is not distributed equally between groups.
- Distorts the apparent effect of an exposure or risk because it is not logically possible to separate the contribution of a single causal factor to an effect, e.g. smoking and alcohol with head and neck cancer.

Confounding variable with examples and their control

A variable that is a known or suspected cause of the outcome under study (or is a surrogate for cause) and is also statistically associated with the exposure of interest is a confounding variable. Formally, a confounding variable may be defined as a variable that is causally related to the condition under study independently of the exposure of primary interest, and is associated with the exposure of primary interest in the study population, but is not a consequence of the exposure. Because of confounding (among other issues), a statistical association between an exposure and a condition does not necessarily mean that the exposure is causally related to the condition. For instance, a statistical association between coffee drinking during pregnancy and an increased likelihood of giving birth to an infant of low birth weight might occur because women who drink coffee are more likely to smoke than non-coffee drinkers.

It is possible that cigarette smoking, not coffee drinking, is the factor that increases the risk for delivery of a low-birth-weight infant.

Confounding is common in observational studies. Rarely are exposures distributed without regard to some aspect of person. In observational studies of the effects of drugs and other therapies, confounding by indication and confounding by severity of illness are particular concerns. Confounding by indication occurs when the provision of a drug or therapy is determined by another factor that is causally related to the outcome of interest, thus distorting the relationship between the therapy and outcome. For example, diuretics are prescribed to treat hypertension. In a study that reported an increased risk of renal cancer in users of diuretics, the possibility that hypertension, the indication for diuretic use, rather than diuretics themselves might be the true risk factor for renal cancer must be considered.

Confounding variables may be taken into account in the study design by matching study subjects on them. Alternatively, confounding variables may be taken into account in data analysis using various statistical procedures. Both matching in the study design and controlling in the analysis are valid ways of taking confounding variables into account. In some instances one can match variables roughly in the study design and then control for them more finely in the analysis.

Careful measurement of confounding variables is important. Unmeasured variables cannot be controlled in the analysis. Mismeasured variables cannot be adequately controlled. For example in finding time duration for wound healing after applying a new drug the confounder is the initial wound size, co-existing illnesses that delay wound healing like diabetes, uraemia, malnutrition etc.

Effect modification

Effect modification, sometimes called statistical interaction, also needs to be considered when studies are designed, analyzed, and interpreted. Effect modification is said to occur when the magnitude of the association between one variable and another differs according to the level of a third variable. For instance, obesity increases the risk for breast cancer in postmenopausal but not premenopausal women; thus, menopausal status is a modifier of the effect of obesity on breast cancer. Asbestos appears to be a stronger risk factor for lung cancer among smokers than among nonsmokers; in other words, smoking modifies the effect of asbestos on lung cancer risk. Detecting effect modification is an important component of the analysis of epidemiologic data.

Bias

Non-random error leads to a deviation of inferences or results from the truth. Any trend in the collection, analysis, interpretation, publication or review of data can lead to conclusions that are systematically different from the truth.

Bias refers to the tendency of a measurement or a statistic to deviate from the true value of the measure or statistic. Bias can arise from many sources and is a common concern in epidemiologic studies. Biases can affect estimates of outcome, of exposure frequency, and of the magnitude of the association between a risk factor and a disease and an intervention or an outcome. As described above, uncontrolled or inadequately controlled confounding can lead to misleading estimates of measures of association. Mismeasurement also has the potential to cause bias.

Information bias is systematic error in measuring the exposure or outcome such that information is more accurate or more complete in one group than another. Examples of information bias include interviewer bias, recall bias, and reporting bias.

Interviewer bias is a systematic error occurring because an interviewer does not gather information in a similar manner in groups being compared. For example, if an interviewer believes, either subconsciously or consciously, that oral contraceptives cause breast cancer, the interviewer might probe more deeply into the oral contraceptive history of cases than of controls.

Recall bias is systematic error resulting from differences in the accuracy or completeness of recall of past events between groups. For example, mothers of infants whose children are born with a congenital malformation may remember events during the pregnancy to a greater extent than mothers of apparently healthy infants.

Reporting bias is a systematic error resulting from the tendency of people in one group to be more or less likely to report information than others. Cases with certain diseases might be more likely to deny that they had used alcohol than controls.

Selection bias is systematic error occurring because of differences between those who are and are not selected for a study or selected to be in a certain group within a study. Ascertainment bias, detection bias, and response bias are generally considered to be types of selection bias.

Ascertainment bias is a systematic error resulting from failure to identify equally all categories of individuals who are supposed to be represented in a group. For instance, a specialty hospital may provide only the sickest of cases to a study and not a representative sample of cases for comparison with controls.

Detection bias is a systematic error resulting from greater likelihood of some cases being identified, diagnosed, or verified than others. For example, pulmonary embolism may be more likely to be detected in women using oral contraceptives than in those not using oral contraceptives because of a greater likelihood of doing a lung scan in oral contraceptive users with chest pain. Thus, an association between use of oral contraceptives and pulmonary embolism might result from the greater likelihood of disease detection in oral contraceptive users rather than from the oral contraceptives themselves.

Response bias is a systematic error occurring because of differences between those who do and do not choose to participate in a study. It also arises because of differences between those who remain in a study and those who are lost-to follow-up. In a cross-sectional study, even when a sample is scientifically selected, if a substantial proportion of those selected decline to participate, the sample is still likely to give biased results. Respondents and non-respondents almost always differ in important ways. If one is trying to learn about the prevalence of a disease, those with serious disease may not be well enough to participate, and those who feel healthy may have little motivation to participate.

If very ill people are unable to come to a clinic to participate in a study, very ill people will be underrepresented as cases in a study. If busy people are less likely than others to be willing to participate as controls in a case-control study, the controls will not be representative of the general population. Similarly, if persons who are sicker are less likely to return for follow-up in a randomized trial, hence, outcome information based on those who return will not be representative of outcomes in all persons who entered the study.

Sampling bias

- Selection of a sample that does not truly represent the population.
- Sampling procedures should be chosen to prevent or minimize bias.

Power of the test

- Probability of correctly rejecting a null hypothesis when it is in fact false; i.e. the probability of finding a specified difference to be statistically significant at a given value.
- Power increases with an increase in sample size.

- Power = 1-beta, and is therefore equal to the probability of a true positive result.

Power can be thought of as the probability that a study will find (or found) a statistically significant difference when, in truth, a difference of a given magnitude exists (or existed). Power is equal to 1-beta (type II error), where beta is the probability of declaring a difference not to be statistically significant when, in truth, a difference exists. The statistical power of a study to detect an effect of given size is determined by its size. Small studies have lower power than larger studies, all other things being equal.

The danger of conducting a study with low statistical power is that a conclusion that an intervention does not work (or that an exposure is not related to disease) will be drawn when, in truth, the intervention works (or the exposure is related to disease). For example, several small studies of intravenous streptokinase in patients with acute myocardial infarction found no statistically significant difference in a post-myocardial infarction outcome between treated and untreated patients. A meta-analysis (Stampfer et al. 1982) and subsequent large study (GISSI 1986) both concluded that streptokinase reduces mortality and reinfarction. The negative findings of initial small studies were a consequence of their small size and low statistical power.

In "negative" studies (i.e. studies that find no effect of the intervention or no association between exposure and disease), the possibility that inadequate statistical power explains the negative result must always be considered. When there are many small studies that are individually statistically insignificant, meta-analysis, may sometimes be a useful way to draw conclusions about the body of literature, overcoming the problem of low statistical power in individual studies. Post hoc estimation of power based on observed results and presentation of 95% confidence limits can put negative findings into perspective. The

Table.6.1   Precision, accuracy, sensitivity, and specificity

Test outcome		Condition present Gold standard	Condition absent Gold standard	
	Test outcome positive	**True positive**	**False positive** (Type I error)	Precision = Σ True positive/ Σ Test outcome positive
	Test outcome negative	**False negative** (Type II error)	**True negative**	Negative predictive value = Σ True negative/ Σ Test outcome negative
		Sensitivity = Σ True positive/ Σ Condition positive	Specificity = Σ True negative/ Σ Condition negative	Accuracy = Σ True positive + Σ True negative/ Σ Total population

careful planning of studies based on a formal sample size calculation is the best way to prevent erroneous conclusions resulting from inadequate statistical power.

Types of data

- Qualitative data – Categorical data
- Quantitative data – Numerical data

Qualitative/Categorical data

There are two types of categorical data:

1. Nominal
2. Ordinal data

1. In nominal data, the variables are divided into named categories. These categories however, cannot be ordered one above another (as they are not greater or lesser than each other).

Example

Nominal data	Categories
Sex/ Gender:	Male, female
Marital status:	Single, married, widowed, Separated, divorced

2. **In ordinal data,** the variables are also divided into a number of categories, but they can be ordered one above another, from lowest to highest or vice versa.

Example: Fair, good, very good, excellent

i. Types of data:

- Primary data (originally collected data)
- Secondary data (after statistical procedures) such as collection, classification, tabulation and presentation.

ii. Collection of primary data:

- Direct personal investigation: the health problems are inquired from the patient.
- (High response rates but costly).
- Indirect personal investigation: The health problems are inquired from other sources.
- Collection through questionnaires and electronic methods
- Collection through enumerators
- Collection through local sources

iii. Collection of secondary data

    a. **Official:** publication of statistical division, ministry of finance, federal and provincial bureaus of statistics.

    b. **Semi-Official**

Research organizations.

    c. **Private Sectors: NGOs.**

Explanation of data analysis

In statistics, *variables* refer to measurable or observable attributes that vary among individuals or over time (e.g. body mass, postoperative complications). *Data* consist of the corresponding measured or observed *values* assumed by these variables under specific conditions (e.g. 70.5 kg, abdominal hematoma). The goal of data analysis is to make statements about the distributional properties of variables, individually or collectively. However, the diverse nature of statistical variables is such that no single analytical method may be applied to all forms of data. As such, understanding the properties of the variables under study is critical to ensure selection of appropriate statistical tests.

All statistical variables may be classified as either *categorical* or *numerical*.

Categorical variables represent *qualitative* observations (e.g. postoperative complications, preoperative diagnosis), whereas numerical variables refer to *quantitative* observations (e.g. body mass, operative time). Generally speaking, numerical data are those whose values are numbers 70.5 kg), whereas categorical data delineate one or more groups (e.g. hematoma, herniation). Numerical variables may be further subdivided into *discrete* and *continuous* types. Discrete variables are those whose values are restricted to a predefined set, typically the integers (e.g. number of revisions). By contrast, continuous variables may assume any intermediate value within a given range (e.g. body mass). These include most clinical measurements, such as weight and length. Statistical data are also frequently categorized according to their *level of measurement* or *data scale*. These two terms are synonymous and refer to the relationships among observable values as restricted by the nature of the measurement system.

Measurement of categorical variables may be either *ordinal*, in which case values have an obvious ordering (e.g. severe pain is greater than moderate pain), or *nominal*, in which no explicit ranking exists (e.g. hematoma versus herniation). All numerical variables prescribe to an innate ordering system, and most are measured along an *interval* scale [the exception being pseudo numerical variables such as cancer staging, where the quantitative differences between values do not reflect magnitudes of effect (e.g. stage one versus stage two versus stage three colon cancer)]. In general, the specific properties of a variable or group of variables (e.g. continuous numerical) will dictate the appropriate statistical measures for their analysis.

TYPES OF BIOSTATISTICS

There are two main types

1. **Descriptive biostatistics:** Deals with the concepts and methods concerned with summarization and description of the important aspects of the numerical data.

2. **Inferential biostatistics:** Deals with procedures for making inferences about the characteristics of the large groups of populations by using a part of the data called the sample population. Formulation of hypothesis, data analysis and reporting statistical significance is an essential part of inferential statistics.

Explanation of biostatistics

in broad terms, analysis of data may be regarded as either descriptive or inferential.

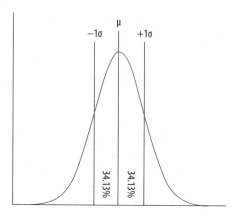

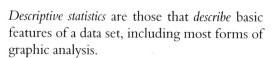

Fig.6.1   Mean in normal distribution curve

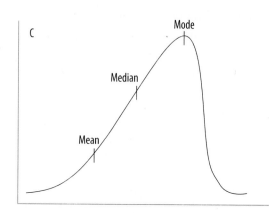

Fig.6.2   Mean, median, and mode

Descriptive statistics are those that *describe* basic features of a data set, including most forms of graphic analysis.

These facilitate identification of patterns and form the basis of nearly every quantitative analysis.

Inferential statistics, by contrast, evaluate relationships among variables (e.g. increased body mass is associated with an increased complication rate).

Treatment of clinical data will typically begin with broad descriptive statistics covering all study data and then proceed to the application of inferential statistics for specific subsets of interest. In their most basic form, descriptive statistics are simply an efficient method of data presentation.

1.   Descriptive statistics

This is particularly important for large data sets, where reporting raw values quickly becomes unavoidable. For categorical data, this is typically achieved through a frequency table, in which the absolute frequencies (i.e. raw counts) or relative frequencies (i.e. fractions of the total) for each group are listed. Common clinical applications include the tabular reporting of complications, risk factors,

and patient demographics. Graphic analysis of categorical data may facilitate comparison of relative frequencies, often in the form of bar graphs or pie charts. Presentation of numerical data requires a more complex descriptive approach. The univariate analysis of the data consists of finding:

a   Central tendency (mean, median, mode)

b   Measure of Dispersion (Range, variance, standard deviation, standard error, confidence intervals)

c   The bivariate analysis and multivariable analysis consist of hypothesis testing and finding values for statistical significance.

a.   Central tendency

Measures of central tendency provide estimates of the "middle" of a data set, and are particularly useful for describing numerical data. These include the familiar metrics of *mean*, *median*, and *mode*. These refer to the arithmetic average, midpoint, and most common values of a set, respectively. Here, "midpoint" signifies the middle value of the ordered set (or the average of the middle two numbers if the sample size is even). Typically, only one of these indicators will be used to

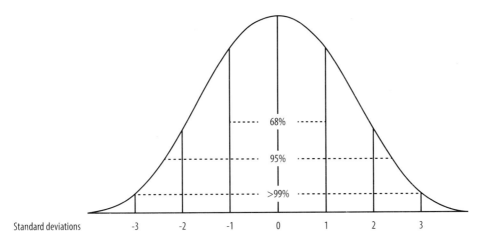

Fig.6.3   Standard deviations

describe any given variable, often dictated by the data scale. The mean is by far the most frequently used measure of central tendency, although specific instances where the median is more appropriate (particularly when dealing with outliers).

The mode is rarely mentioned by name, but it is nearly ubiquitous in any discussion of categorical data (e.g. "the most common...," "the majority...").

b.   Measures of dispersion

Dispersion refers to the spread of the values around the central tendency (typically, the mean).

The *range* is the most simple measure of dispersion, defined as the difference between the highest and lowest values in a set. For data that are interval in nature, a more accurate and detailed estimate is provided by the *variance*, which measures how closely individual values cluster around the mean. The *SD*, defined as the square root of the variance, provides an estimate for the typical distance of a value from the mean. Another related measure commonly used to describe the behavior of a variable is the

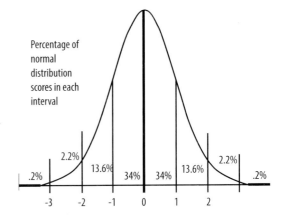

Fig.6.4   Percentage of normal distribution scores in each interval

skewness, which evaluates the symmetry of data relative to their mean. Together, these metrics provide a concise numerical description of the distribution of values throughout a data set.

$$Z = x \text{ eq } x), \sigma)$$

c.   Statistical distributions

The relationships observed among measures of central tendency and dispersion frequently

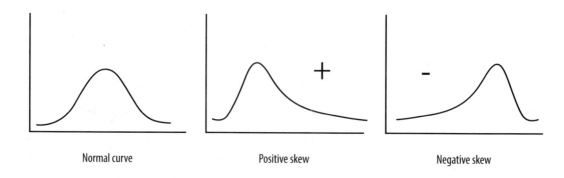

Fig.6.5   Normal curve and skewness

follow specific well-characterized patterns, which may be described mathematically in the form of statistical distributions. The most common of these is the *normal distribution*, which corresponds to a symmetric, bell-shaped curve. This distribution has several important and unique properties, including identical values of the mean, median, and mode. Moreover, a normal distribution implies that approximately 68, 95, and 99.7 percent of all values will fall within 1, 2, and 3 SD of the mean, respectively. In general, the mean is the preferred measure of central tendency for symmetrical (e.g. normal) distributions; however, it is strongly influenced by outliers and can thus be misleading in skewed distributions. The median typically provides a more reliable metric for heavily or predictably skewed distributions. Although most clinical data can usually be characterized by a normal distribution, several variables such as length of stay and body mass may be predictably skewed (e.g. both frequently exhibit positive skewness because of unbalanced outliers on the upper end).

Graphic analyses such as Q-Q plots and histograms are often helpful for evaluating deviations from normality, and more sophisticated computational methods have also been developed. When identified, non-normal data can occasionally be mathematically transformed to adopt a normal distribution (e.g. using the variable's logarithm, square root, or multiplicative inverse). This is strongly preferable where possible, as normality permits the use of highly specific *parametric tests*, which use knowledge of the underlying data distribution to more precisely evaluate significance. Analysis of non-normally distributed data requires a separate, more general class of statistical methods; incorrectly applying normality-based tests to these data will yield inaccurate results.

2.   Inferential statistics

Where descriptive statistics describe basic features of a data set (e.g. mean body mass), statistical inference makes claims about the nature and relationships of the underlying variables that give rise to the observed data (e.g. "increased body mass leads to an increased incidence of hematomas"). This process is critically dependent on the ability to distinguish true relationships from random variation, and rigorous numerical analysis is often required to achieve this end.

a. Standard error

Generally speaking, any collection of observed data represents only a small subset of all the data that *could* be observed for that variable under similar conditions. As such, a variable's distribution *within* a given data set is merely a sampling of the true behavior of that variable. By assuming that the degree of variance exhibited by the observed data is approximately that of the true variable, it is possible to estimate the sampling error associated with each variable under study. For example, consider intercanthal measurements of 10 adults with Apert syndrome. This is a small sample relative to all affected adults and, as such, repeating these measurements for another 10 patients would be expected to yield a different mean distance. The degree to which this sample mean will vary on repeated measurements can be estimated based on the variance within the (initial) observed data.

The resulting quantity, termed the *standard error of the mean (SEM)*, is frequently used as a measure of the reliability of a data set.

$$SEM = \frac{SD}{\sqrt{n}}$$

b. Confidence intervals

Confidence intervals provide another index of the reliability of a sample mean, denoting numerical limits within which a given variable is expected to occur. These limits may be adjusted to encompass any fraction of expected outcomes but are typically defined using the 95 percent threshold (i.e. with specific error tolerance = 0.05). When the data can be assumed to follow a normal distribution, confidence intervals may be quickly computed using the SEM as a measure of the true SD (within 2 of which 95 percent of normally distributed data fall). Here, the 95 percent confidence interval is simply the mean 2 + SEM. However, as described above, if the true distribution is unknown, the SEM is often an unreliable estimator. For such cases, a more robust interval may be obtained using other methods, as described by Efron and Tibshirani.

In certain situations, confidence intervals may also be used to evaluate statistical significance. This is most commonly achieved by computing the confidence intervals for two variables and demonstrating that they do or do not overlap. For example, consider the 95 percent confidence intervals for mean artery diameter (6.2 + 1.1 mm) and vein diameter (8.9 + 1.3 mm). Because these two intervals (5.1 to 7.3 mm and 7.6 to 10.2 mm) do not overlap, this indicates a statistically significant difference with $p < 0.05$.

c. Hypothesis testing

Hypothesis testing is the most common and most general form of statistical inference. This process is centered around the generation of a *null hypothesis*, which serves as the predicate for subsequent evaluation. The essence of hypothesis testing is to specify a proposition (before data collection) and then use the sample data to disprove it. This process typically proceeds through several general stages, including computation of a *p* value, which represents a decreasing index of reliability for the null hypothesis. Although an explicit statement of the null hypothesis is often omitted, it is implicit in declaring that a given difference is "statistically significant with $p < 0.05$" that the null hypothesis of "no difference exists" is rejected at a threshold of 0.05.

There is always a level of uncertainty associated with accepting (or rejecting) the null hypothesis. An incorrect rejection (i.e. concluding that a difference exists, when in fact one does not) is referred to as a *type I error*, the probability of which is equal to the *p* value. A *type II error* describes the failure to reject a faulty null hypothesis (i.e. not finding a difference, when one actually exists).

Table.6.2   Type I and type II errors

True Situation	Decision	
	Accept H_o	Reject H_o
H_o is true	Correct decision (No error)	Wrong decision (Type I error)α - error
H_o is false	Wrong decision (Type II error) β-error	Correct decision (No error)

The *power* of a study is defined as the probability of *not* making a type II error; that is, the likelihood of detecting a statistically significant difference when one actually exists. This is dependent on the sample size and significance threshold (p), and the extent of true difference. When designing a clinical study, a *power analysis* is frequently used to determine the minimum sample size required to achieve an acceptable rate of type II error. These computations are heavily distribution dependent, and their specific formulae are available on softwares. The cross-sectional studies, case-control and cohort studies can be calculated at 95% CI, and 80% power of test using EPI-inf 2000 software. The sample calculations of experimental studies can be done using 95% CI and effect size by software Raosoft.

Steps in hypothesis testing

1. Formulate a Hypothesis.
2. Specify the level of significance.
3. Select the appropriate statistical test.
4. Compute the value of the statistical test.
5. Compute the value of p.
6. Accept or reject Hypothesis.

Hypothesis testing

- Null vs. Alternative hypothesis.
- Null hypothesis is any hypothesis which

is to be tested for possible rejection under the assumption that it is true.

- It usually contains a term "no effects".

Example

There is no difference between two teaching methods.

- **Level of significance (α)**

  It is a probability to reject the null hypothesis when it is true.

  We usually set 5%.

  It may be 1% or 10%, (researcher's choice).

- **Significance value (p-value)**

  Calculated probability

  Significant, if less than selected (α)

- **Type I vs. Type II error**

  Type I error (rejecting H_0 when it is true)

  It is also called ALPHA (level of significance).

  It should be as minimum as possible.

  Type II error (accepting H_0 when it is wrong)

  It is also called BETA (Power of the test).

Statistical tests

Selecting an appropriate statistical test is critical for accurate data analysis. Determining the optimal method for a given data set must take into account several factors, chief among which are the limitations (e.g. continuous versus discrete) and distributional properties (e.g. normal versus skewed) of the variables under study.

Statistical tests for categorical data

For comparisons among categorical variables, the null hypothesis typically states that the distribution of one variable is independent from those of the other variables (i.e. no relationship exists).

Statistical tests, then, evaluate whether the observed frequencies of joint occurrences differ from the products of the individual observed frequencies for each variable (i.e. the expected overlap for independent distributions). *Pearson's Chi square test* is the most commonly used method and may be applied to the majority of categorical data. For example, to evaluate the association between diabetes and post-operative infection, a Chi square test would compare the observed incidence of post-operative infections in diabetic patients with that otherwise expected, based on the observed frequencies of the remaining category pairs (e.g. postoperative infections in non-diabetics, diabetics without post-operative infections). When the expected number of co-occurrences for any pair is very small, *Fisher's exact test* offers a nonparametric alternative for statistical analysis.

Statistical tests for numerical data

Analysis of numerical variables typically takes the form of either correlation or regression analysis.

Where the former simply evaluates the degree of relationship among variables, regression analysis seeks to formalize this relationship as a mathematical model. In deciding which form of analysis is more appropriate, it is helpful to distinguish between *independent* (predictive)

variables and *dependent* (predicted) variables. Typically, dependent variables represent measured endpoints (e.g. complications), whereas independent variables are those hypothesized to influence these endpoints (e.g. body mass).

Correlation analysis is typically used to evaluate the degree of associations among large numbers of independent variables without establishing causal relationships. The most common method is *Pearson's correlation* (r), which measures the linear dependence of normally distributed numerical variables. This test assigns an r value to the degree of correlation, ranging from –1 to 1, with 0 representing no correlation and +1/–1 corresponding to perfect correlation / anticorrelation. When the assumption of normality cannot be made, *Spearman's rank correlation coefficient ()* provides a nonparametric alternative to Pearson's correlation.

Both measures are typically reported in conjunction with a p value, representing the likelihood of observing a relationship of such strength by random chance; however, it is important to note that this p value itself does not represent the degree of the association and thus should function only as a means of validating large correlation coefficients.

For example, Pearson's correlation could be used to evaluate the fidelity of automated blood pressure readings compared with physician-administered measurements, where a correlation coefficient of one may correspond either to perfect agreement or perfectly reproducible error (e.g. the automated reading is always exactly three higher than that of the physician).

Regression analysis is more appropriate to evaluate the specific relationship between a dependent variable and one or more independent variables. The most familiar application involves the comparison of two variables through *linear regression analysis*; that is, for independent variable x and dependent

Table.6.3   Selection of statistical tests

Parametric	Non-parametric
T- Value:	Chi- square test ($\chi 2$)
One sample, paired and unpaired t-tests	
Z-Value: z test	Fisher's test
	U- value: Mann-Whitney test
	Wilcoxon rank sum
	Mcnemar test
Advance statistical hypothesis tests	
Repeated measures ANOVA	
One way ANOVA	
Two way ANOVA	
Post hoc analysis	
ANCOVA	
MANOVA	
Simple and multiple linear regression	
Logistic regression	
Survival analyses	
Nonlinear regression	

variable y, determining the optimal linear equation (i.e. y _ a _ b _ x) to fit the set of observed data pairs {x, y}. Such analyses are frequently accompanied by a scatterplot, which illustrates the observed distribution of data pairs relative to the best linear fit. Although less intuitive, linear regression analysis may be similarly extended to interrogate any number of independent variables (i.e. y _ m1 _ x1 _ m2 _ x2 _...)

When more complex, nonlinear relationships exist between variables, the data may occasionally be transformed (e.g. substituting the variable's natural logarithm) to establish a linear relationship; otherwise, more elaborate

techniques such as *logistic regression analysis* may be required.

Statistical tests for mixed categorical and numerical data

When comparing categorical data with numerical data, it is again important to distinguish between *independent* and *dependent* variables. Statistical analyses of independent numerical and dependent categorical data focus on developing mathematical classifiers based on one or more numerical variables to predict the outcome of the (dependent) categorical variable. These methods are frequently used to evaluate diagnostic and therapeutic implications (e.g. "prostate-specific antigen < 6.0 is associated with a 35 percent risk of prostate cancer"); however, the computational complexity of these *discriminant analyses* grows quickly with the number of variables and generally requires more sophisticated mathematical software, for which consultation with a biostatistician with the necessary resources is advised. The analysis of dependent discrete data with independent continuous data is more broad in scope, with distinct approaches based on the specific properties of the dependent data. The most simple comparisons consist of one independent categorical variable and one dependent numerical variable. These will typically involve two groups of data (i.e. one discrete variable with two possible values, such as treatment versus control). This requires a two sample *t* test, which may be either *paired* or *unpaired*.

The unpaired *t* test is the more common of the two and may be applied for the majority of comparisons. The paired *t* test is only necessary when the independent variable distinguishes between two interdependent measurements. For example, when comparing the healing properties of two wounds on opposite sides of the same mouse, one treated with a dressing and the other a "control," the independent variable (treatment status) does not fully disjoin the dependent variables (rate of healing) on individual mice. A paired *t* test is required to make the necessary statistical adjustments in such cases. In addition, each *t* test may also be *one-tailed* or *two-tailed*, depending on whether experimental deviations are restricted to one direction.

Nearly all clinical analyses should use a two tailed test, with a one-tailed test used only for situations where differences in one direction or the other are not merely unexpected but impossible.

Analysis of variance is a generalized version of the two-sample *t* test that permits comparisons of more than two groups (i.e. a discrete variable with more than two possible values). Analysis of variance may be either, *one-way* or *two-way*, similar to the unpaired and paired forms of the *t* test. *Factorial analysis of variance* may be used to evaluate the effects of more than one independent variable, and *multivariate analysis of variance* is used to study more than one dependent variable. All *t* tests, and even the more general analysis of variance, are based on the assumption that the underlying variables obey a normal distribution. In situations where the assumption of normality is not valid, nonparametric alternative tests must be used. Although more robust, these nonparametric tests have less statistical power than their parametric counterparts and are thus avoided where possible.

Summary of parametric and non-parametric methods

There are parametric methods of hypothesis testing appropriate to parametric data (numerical measures) and nonparametric methods hypothesis testing appropriate to nonparametric data (ordinal or nominal measures).

Making an appropriate choice for statistical methods depends mainly on:

Data measures type (numerical, nominal or ordinal)

Independent or related (pared) samples

Sample size (n>30 or n<30)

Number of groups (one, two or more)

Directional or non-directional research question in terms of statistical hypotheses

Data Distribution type (normal or skewed)

Homogeneity of variance

Comparing means in two groups with the t-test

Actually we can use the t-test under the conditions:

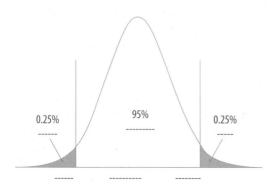

Fig.6.6 Normal distribution curve

1. The data should follow the normal distribution

2. Homogeneity of variance (the population variance are equal)

3. Numerical measures of data. Continuous data sets are present

4. Having no more than two groups

If the data do not respect these conditions you should rather apply non-parametric tests:

The t statistic for testing the mean difference in two independent groups has the difference between the means in the numerator and the standard error of the mean difference in the denominator; in symbols it is:

t-observed = Mean difference/difference of SEM

t–observed (for comparing to critical value—t-table)

D–mean difference;

SEM—standard of the mean error difference;

Draw and state the conclusions.

After performing the calculation of t-observed we have to find the t-tabel (critical value) from the special table in order to compare it:

If t-observed is larger than the critical value the null hypothesis is rejected such the test result is said the difference between the compared means to be statistically significant.

If t-observed is less then critical value the null hypothesis is not rejected such the test result is said the difference between the compared means to be not statistically significant.

Critical value (t-table)

If the numbers of observations "n" >120 then the critical value is already known: t = 1.96 (when); t = 2.58 (when); t = 3.29 (when).

If the numbers of observations "n" < 120 then the critical value is taken from the special table, according to their degrees freedom which are defined as (n1+n2 -2).

Different situations in normal distribution data analysis

1. Comparison of one group with a standard value: One sample t-test

2. Comparison of two groups:

   o Independent sample t-test

   o Dependent sample t-test

3. Comparison of three groups: Analysis of variance (ANOVA).

The detailed description of each test with examples is as follows:

One sample t-test

The one sample t-test is used to comparing a continuous data with a standard given value.

- Always check for following assumptions before applying one sample t-test.

  i.   The data should be continuous.

  ii. The data should be taken at random (probability sampling).

  iii. The data should follow a normal distribution.

  iv. The sample size should be adequate.

Formula: One sample t-test:

$$t = \frac{\overline{X} - \mu_0}{s/\sqrt{n}}$$

μ = mean of population

$\overline{X}$ = X bar is mean of sample

S = standard deviation

n = sample size

Example

Mean height of girls of 18 years in Lahore is 160 cm. In university XYZ, mean height of girls of 18 years is found to be 164 cm. The statistical significance will be tested by one sample t-test in this scenario where obtained value of data set is compared with standard value.

Independent sample t-test

- Situation

$$t = (\overline{x}_1 - \overline{x}_2) / s \sqrt{\frac{1}{n_1} + \frac{1}{n_2}}$$

  o It compares two independent groups on the basis of their means.

- Assumptions.
  o Data should be continuous.
  o Data should be taken at random.
  o Both groups should follow a normal distribution.
  o Both groups should be independent.

S = standard deviation

n_1 = sample size in group1

n_2 = sample size in group2

χ_1 = mean in group1

χ_2 = mean in group2

Example: Pulse rates in two groups consisting of males and females were observed. The total number of males was n_1. The total number of females was n_2. Mean pulse rate in males was $\square_1$. Mean pulse rate in females was $\square_2$. The two groups had equal variance. The standard deviation was S. The distribution of data was normal. The difference in means was calculated and a t-test was computed to

Table.6.4   Selection of statistical tests

Level of training	n	S²	$\square$
Advanced	10	24.2	21.54
Intermediate	10	27.1	18.64
Beginner	10	30.2	17.76

find out the difference in the two groups was statistically significant.

Paired sample t-test (dependent sample t-test)

- Situation
  o When we get information twice from the same individual
  o When we take data in crossover design
  o When our data is correlated with each other

- Assumptions
  o Data should be continuous and taken at random.
  o Difference in data should be normally distributed.

Example

Pulse rate of 30 students before and after exercise

Analysis of variance (ANOVA)

- Situation
  o It is used to compare the mean of more than two groups.

Table.6.5   Selection of statistical tests

Source	df	SS	MS	F value
Treatments	2	180.067	90.033	4.662
Error	27	521.46	19.313	
Total	29	702.527		

- Assumptions
  - o Data should be continuous
  - o Data should be taken at random
  - o Data should be normally distributed
- All the groups should be independent.

Example

A researcher wishes to determine whether the mean times required to complete a certain task differ for the three levels of student's training. He randomly selected 10 students with each of the three levels of training (beginners, intermediate and advanced). Do the data provide sufficient evidence to indicate that the mean times required to complete a certain task differ for at least two of the three levels of training? The data is summarized in the table.

Where:

N = number of students

$\square$ = mean of group

S = standard deviation

H_a: The mean times required to complete a certain task differ for at least two of the three levels of training.

H_o: The mean times required to complete a certain task do not differ the three levels of training. $(\mu_B = \mu_I = \mu_A)$

Assumptions: The samples were drawn independently and randomly from the three populations. The time required to complete the task is normally distributed for each of the three levels of training. The populations have equal variances.

Decision: Reject H_o.

Conclusion:

There is sufficient evidence to indicate that the mean times required to complete a certain task differ for at least two of the three levels of training.

Analysis of covariance

a. Introduction

The Analysis of Covariance (generally known as ANCOVA) is a technique that sits between analysis of variance and regression analysis. It has a number of purposes but the two that are, perhaps, of most importance are:

i. To increase the precision of comparisons between groups by accounting to

   variation on important prognostic variables.

ii. To "adjust" comparisons between groups for imbalances in important prognostic variables between these groups.

The second purpose is one that is new in ANCOVA, the first being a purpose shared by many techniques, specifically simple linear regression. Another reason to concentrate on point 2 is that "adjustments" for other variables, or "adjusted means" or "adjusted relative risks" are often encountered in medical literature. Whether relative risks, hazard rates or simply means are adjusted depends on whether the outcome measurement is, respectively, binary/categorical, survival data or continuous. The following example is based on an outcome that is taken to be continuous, because it is easier

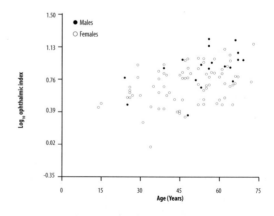

Fig.6.7 Plot of $\log_{10}$ against age, with sex of patient

to demonstrate the ideas behind "adjustment" with this type of outcome. Nevertheless the underlying ideas are the same for all types of outcome.

The example concerns thyroid-associated ophthalmopathy. The data are from the first visit of each of 101 patients made to a combined thyroid-eye clinic. For our purposes we will consider only three of several variables measured, namely the age of the patient, the sex of the patient and the ophthalmic index (OI) which is a composite score measuring several aspects of ophthalmic performance, the larger the value of OI, the poorer the performance. Preliminary analysis suggested the analysis be based on the log the OI. More details of the study can be found in Perros *et al. Clinical Endocrinology*, 1993, **38,** 367-372. As with most statistical techniques, the availability of software means that it is not necessary to know the numerical procedures needed in order to use ANCOVA, so most emphasis will be placed on understanding the approach behind the method.

b. The data and the problem

Interest surrounds whether the OI is worse for men or women. Superficially this can be answered by looking at the means in the two groups. Some summary statistics are:

Sample size mean log10 OI (SD)

Male 20 0.885 (0.218)

Female 81 0.699 (0.215)

Thus it appears that the ophthalmic performance of the men is worse. Indeed, this is confirmed by a *t*-test, which gives P = 0.0008 and a 95% confidence interval for the difference in log OI (males - females) of 0.08, 0.29. However, before concluding that this analysis is all that is needed it is, as ever, wise to plot the data.

i. Males clearly have larger values of the OI.

ii. The ophthalmic index deteriorates with age.

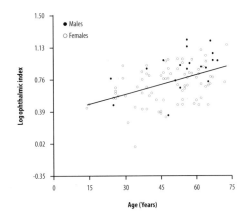

Fig.6.8   Regression of $\log_{10}$ on age, P<0.001

iii. There is a suggestion that the male patients may be older than the female patients.

If these observations are correct the preceding analysis is unreliable because the apparently larger OI in males may not reflect a difference between the sexes *per se* but simply that OI is larger in older patients and in this sample the males are older than the females. ANCOVA is a technique which attempts to make allowance for imbalances between groups and in this instance would try to determine whether there is a difference between the sexes in OI, independent of any age differences between the sexes that may exist.

The mean ages in the men and women are rather different, as the following table shows:

Sample size mean age (yrs.) (SD)

Male 20 53.8 (12.8)

Female 81 48.2 (13.5)

A formal hypothesis test gives $t = 1.70$, P = 0.09 with 95% confidence interval for the difference in means, male - female, of -1.0, 12.3. Although there is no conclusive evidence of an age difference between the groups, this analysis certainly does not rule out this possibility. It may be, e.g. that there really is a difference in the ages of male and female patients with thyroid-associated eye disease

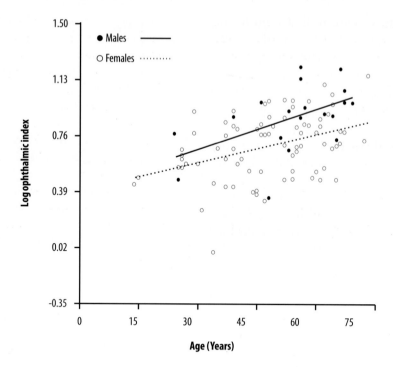

Fig.6.9   Separate regression lines for males and females

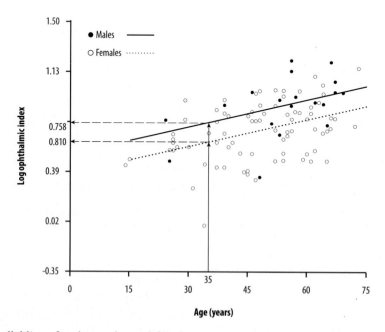

Fig.6.10   Parallel lines fitted to males and females

but because there were only 20 males in the sample the test lacked the power to attain nominal levels of statistical significance. From this analysis it is important to realise that an age difference may exist and be sufficiently large to render any conclusion on the sex difference in OI unsafe unless some account is taken of age in the analysis.

3. Taking account of age

That age and log OI are related is confirmed by a simple regression analysis.

Figure 2 shows the relation between age and log OI and the accompanying regression line indicates quantitatively how the mean log OI changes with age. The idea behind ANCOVA is to extend this type of analysis: if differences in log OI due to age can be predicted then the differences in log OI between males and females that would be expected due to the age difference between these groups can also be predicted. Any difference between males and females beyond this prediction cannot be put down to differences in age. This is achieved by fitting separate regression lines to males and females. However, for reasons that will become apparent this has to be done in a special way as the fitted lines in the males and females must be parallel. If a regression line is fitted to the females and another one to the males, then the position in figure 3 would generally obtain, with the fitted lines not being parallel.

Using a method, the details of which need not concern us, it is possible to fit a pair of regression lines, one for males and one for females, that are constrained to be parallel: (this method is essentially ANCOVA although in routine use it is not usual for the graph of the parallel lines to be displayed, indeed finding their equations from the output is not straightforward). When this is done the result is as in figure 4.

Two questions arise: First, how does this help us to "adjust" for sex differences and second,

is it legitimate to fit parallel lines in this way? The answer to the first point is embodied in the graph. As an example consider a 35-year-old patient, then the expected log OI is shown on the graph: if the patient is female it is 0.610, whereas for a male it is 0.758. The difference between these, 0.758-0.610 = 0.148, is the mean difference in log OI between males and females aged 35. However, because the regression lines are parallel, this difference is the same whatever the age of the patient. Consequently the mean sex difference, *adjusted for age* is simply the vertical difference between the lines. Any hypothesis test for a sex difference, adjusting for age, amounts to testing whether the sample provides evidence that the distance between the lines is zero or not. The adjustment for age arises because a method for modelling age has been incorporated into a comparison of males and females. The adjustment· is, strictly, only for the *difference* between the sexes and from figure 4 there is no obvious definition of the adjusted mean log OI for men and for women. A method, albeit rather arbitrary, that is often used is to find the mean log OI from figure 4 using not age 35, but the mean age in the combined sample, which is 49.3 years, giving:

adjusted mean log OI (males) = 0.854 adjusted mean log OI (females) = 0.707. These are the figures that the ANCOVA command will report. The second problem mentioned above, namely whether the analyst is entitled to fit parallel lines, is important but often rather neglected in discussions of ANCOVA. Only a few general remarks will be made here.

i.   Clearly in most analyses the only justification for any statistical model is that it fits the data, and it may be that two non-parallel straight lines fit the data far better than two parallel lines. In the present example the separate lines in figure 3, are not far from parallel and the deviation from parallelism may be due to sampling error.

ii. If parallel lines cannot be fitted then it is

impossible to report a single adjusted sex difference, as the vertical distance between the lines will change depending on the age of the patient. It must then be admitted that the method loses much of its appeal.

iii. In practice several options are available. A formal significance test of non-parallelism can be performed. If non-parallelism is a problem then some transformation of the response may be helpful.

4. Summary of analysis of covariance

The method of ANCOVA allows the analyst to make comparisons between groups that are not comparable with respect to some important variable, often referred to as a covariate. This is done by making an adjustment based on fitting a particular kind of regression line. When the imbalance between the groups is not large this method may be very helpful, however it is worth bearing in mind that the "adjustment" is done through a particular statistical model and it may be unwise to rely on such a device to bring into balance two highly divergent groups. In addition to allowing for imbalances, the method removes variation due to the covariate and therefore provides a more precise analysis. A geometrical interpretation is that the 'unexplained variation' with respect to which the significances of group differences are ultimately assessed is the variation about the lines in figure 4, whereas an analysis ignoring the covariate would use the variation about the group means, which will clearly be greater.

5. Correlation techniques

Correlation is used to establish and quantify the strength and direction of the relationship between two variables. The strength of the relationship is indicated by the size of the coefficient whereas its direction is indicated by the sign. A plus sign means positive correlation and minus sign means negative correlation. If there is no relationship between two variables then the coefficient will be zero. Coefficient beyond 0.5 are regarded as strong and less than 0.5 are regarded as weak associations.

Pearson's correlation coefficient

Pearson's correlation coefficient is one measure of the relationship between two *numerical* characteristics, symbolized by "X" and "Y". The correlation coefficient is denoted by "r", it is calculated using the formula:

$$r =$$

The correlation coefficient is a dimensionless number (no units of measurement). The maximum values that "r" can achieve is 1, and its minimum values is -1. Therefore, for any given set data: -1 r 1

Coefficient of correlation interpretation is based on the relation noted above:

Positively correlation (+), when coefficient of correlation is 0 r 1 : "Y" tends to increase in magnitude as "X" increases;

Negatively correlation (-), when coefficient of correlation is -1 r 0 : "Y" decreases as "X" incleases;

The values r = 1 and r = -1 occur when there is exact linear relationship between X and Y, if r = 0 means no linear relationship or no correlation exists between two variables.

There are following crude rules for ***interpreting the size of correlation:***

The correlation coefficient equal one denote a perfect linear and ***strong relationship;***

Correlations from 0 to 0.25 (or – 0.25) indicate *little or no relationship*;

Correlations from 0.25 to 0.50 (or -0.25 to – 0.50) indicate ***a fair degree of relationship;***

Correlations from 0.50 to 0.75 (or – 0.50 to – 0.75) indicate ***a good relationship***;

Correlations greater than 0.75 (or – 0.75) indicate ***a very good to excellent relationship.***

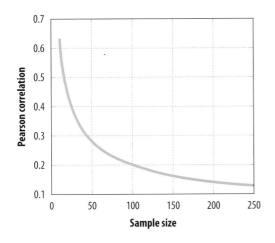

Fig.6.11 Pearson's correlation and sample size estimations

Note that correlation does not imply causation; there is only a measure of straight-line relationship.

Sometimes the correlation is squared (r2) to form a useful statistic called the **coefficient of determination** or **r-squared:**

It is a statistical term that tells us how good one variable is at predicting another.

r2 = 1.0 means given value of one variable can perfectly predict the value for other variable.

r2 = 0 means knowing either variable does not predict the other variable.

The higher r2 value means more correlation is there between two variables. Though coefficient of determination is denoted the common association of the factors that influence the two variables. In other words, the coefficient of determination indicates the part of total value dispersion of variable can be explained or justified by dispersion of the values of the other variable. Sometimes coefficient of determination is presented in percent, being multiplied by 100.

Spearman's rank correlation coefficient

Like other parametric techniques Pearson's correlation coefficient is very sensitive to outlying values. Instead of that the Spearman's rank correlation is used when one or both of the relevant variables are ordinal (or one ordinal and one numerical) characteristics and when the numerical observations are skewed with extreme values.

Table 6.6 One way table

Correlation

[Data Set3] c: \ User\ Stephanic\ Download \ 216 data. sav

Correlation		Number of older siblings	Grade point average
Number of older siblings	Pearson's correlation	1	-098
	Sig. (1-tailed)		.259
	N		46
Grade Point Average	Pearson correlation	-098	1
	Sig. (1-tailed)	.259	
	N	46	46

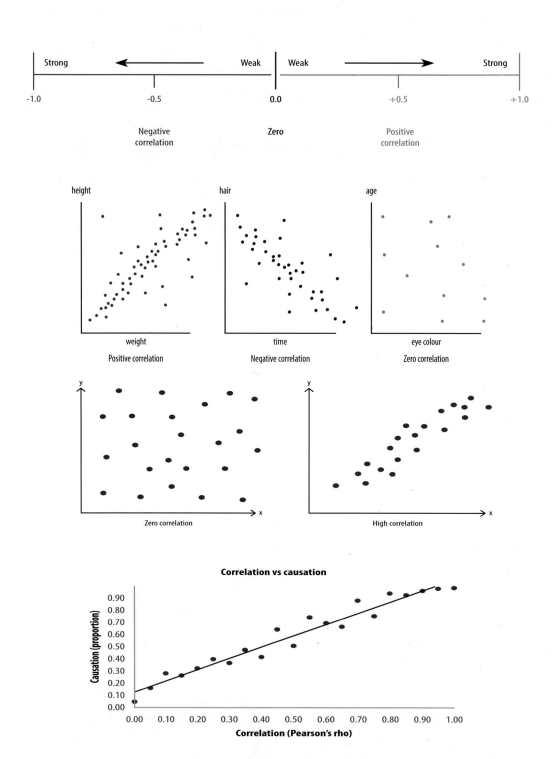

Fig.6.12   Correlation coefficient shows strength and direction of correlation

Table 6.7   Parametric and non-parametric tests

Parametric	Non-Parametric
One sample t-test	Sign test/Wilcoxon signed rank test
Paired t-test	Sign test/Wilcoxon signed rank test
2 Sample t-test	Mann Whitney U-test/ Wilcoxon signed rank test
Anova	Kruskal Wall test

Sourte: Chan Y.N. Biostatistics 102: Quantitative data-parametric and non-parametric tests, singapore med, 2003 Vol 44 (8): 391396

The calculation of the Spearman rank correlation, symbolized as rs involves rank ordering the values on each of the characteristics from lower to highest; the ranks are then treated, as they were the actual values themselves.

As the Pearson's correlation coefficient, the Spearman rank correlation coefficient ranges in value from -1 to 1. Values of rs close to the extremes indicate a high degree of correlation between X and Y; values near 0 imply a lack of linear association between the two variables.

Pearson's correlation coefficient

   o   Spearman's   rank   correlation coefficient

A lot of medical researches are related to relationship between two or more characteristics. For this kind of purpose it is appropriate to use correlation that is able to examining the relationship between two variables.

Non-parametric tests

Chi-squares test

Chi-Square test is employed to determine if there is an *association between categorical variables*.

When the word *association* is used in the statistical sense, a comparison is implied.

Formula for calculating chi-square value:

$$c^2 = å\ (O - E)^2 / E$$

O is the observe frequency (indicated in the table).

E is the expected frequency to be calculated.

å (the sum of) add together the products of $(O-E)2$ for all the cell of the table.

For two by two tables (which contain four cells) the formula is.

$$\chi^2 = (O_1-\Sigma_1)^2 /\Sigma_1 + (O_2 - \Sigma_2)^2 / \Sigma_2 + (O_3 - \Sigma_3)^2 / \Sigma_3 + (O_4 - \Sigma_4)^2/\Sigma_4.$$

Where

$\chi^2 =$ Chi square

$å =$ Summation

$O =$ Observed value

$\Sigma =$ Expected value

Non-parametric tests

1. McNemar's test

2. Fisher exact test

3. Mantel-Haenszel test

4. Sign test

5. Wilcoxon rank-sum test

6. Mann-Whitney U test

7. Kruskal-Wallis test

8. F-test

Multivariable analysis

Multivariable analysis is a tool for determining the relative contributions of different causes to a single event.

Multivariable   analysis   means   multiple

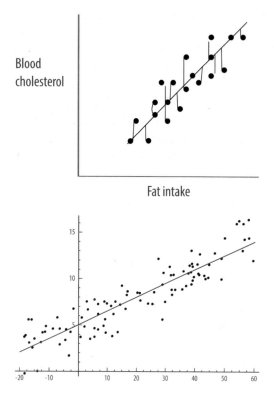

Fig.6.13   Graphs of regression analysis

For example

Researcher studied the risk factors of pregnancy induced hypertension. The risk factors (independent variables) identified were maternal age above 30 years, family history of hypertension and diet rich in salt and fats. The Hosmer-Lemeshow Model showed good fit for logistic regression. The various independent variables were found associated with pregnancy induced hypertension after removing the confounders through analysis by logistic regression. The p value less than 0.05 was considered significant.

Uses of multivariable models in medicine

The common uses of multivariable models are:

1. Identify prognostic factors while adjusting for potential confounders

2. Adjust for differences in baseline characteristics

3. Determine prognosis (prognostic models)

4. Determine diagnosis (diagnostic models)

variables are used to predict a single outcome e.g. linear regression, logistic regression etc.

Regression analysis

It is used to express the functional relationship between two variables so that the value of one variable can be predicted from the knowledge of the other.

Linear regression: The Linear regression model is used when the increase in independent variables causes the increase in mean or expected value of outcome in a linear fashion or vice versa.

Logistic regression: The Logistic regression model is used to compare the estimated probability of outcome to the observed probability of outcome.

Steps for constructing a multivariable model

Step1: Perform univariate statistics to understand distribution of the variables. Mean, standard deviations, standard errors should be calculated. Normal distribution, skewed distribution and outliers should be identified.

Step2: Perform bivariate analysis of independent variables against outcome variable.

Step3: The nominal independent variables should be transformed into multiple dichotomous variables.

Step4: Assess whether the data fit the assumptions of multivariable model (linearity, normal distribution, equal variance) on a bivariate basis. Transform or group any

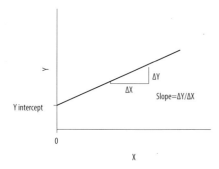

Fig.6.14   Graph of multivariable analysis

variables that show significant bivariate departures from the assumptions of the model.

Step5: Run a correlation matrix. If any pair of independent variables are correlated at >0.90 multicollinearity, decide one to keep and one to exclude.

Step6: Assess how much missing data is present in multivariable analysis.

Step7: Perform the multivariable analysis with dependent and independent variables.

Step8: Perform an assessment of fit of the model and its ability to predict the outcome for study subjects.

Statistical models in multivariable analysis

Most regression models are described in terms of the way the outcome variable is modeled: in linear regression the outcome is continuous; logistic regression has a dichotomous outcome, and survival analysis involves a time to event outcome. Statistically speaking, multivariate analysis refers to statistical models that have two or more dependent or outcome variables, and multivariable analysis refers to statistical models in which there are multiple independent or response variables.

A multivariable model can be thought of as a model in which multiple variables are found on the right side of the model equation. This

type of statistical model can be used to attempt to assess the relationship between a number of variables; one can assess independent relationships while adjusting for potential confounders.

A simple linear regression model has a continuous outcome and one predictor, whereas a multiple or multivariable linear regression model has a continuous outcome and multiple predictors (continuous or categorical). A simple linear regression model would have the form

$$y = \alpha + x\beta + \varepsilon$$

(1)

By contrast, a multivariable or multiple linear regression model would take the form:

$$y = \alpha + x1\beta1 + x2\beta2 + \ldots + xk\beta k + \varepsilon$$

(2)

where y is a continuous dependent variable, x is a single predictor in the simple regression model, and x_1, x_2, ..., x_k are the predictors in the multivariable model.

As is the case with linear models, logistic and proportional hazards regression models can be simple or multivariable. Each of these model structures has a single outcome variable and one or more independent or predictor variables.

Multivariate, by contrast, refers to the modelling of data that are often derived from longitudinal studies, wherein an outcome is measured for the same individual at multiple time points (repeated measures), or the modelling of nested/clustered data, wherein there are multiple individuals in each cluster. A multivariate linear regression model would have the form:

$$Yn \times p = Xn \times (k+1)\beta(k+1) \times p + \varepsilon$$

(3)

where the relationships between multiple dependent variables (i.e. Ys)—measures of multiple outcomes—and a single set of

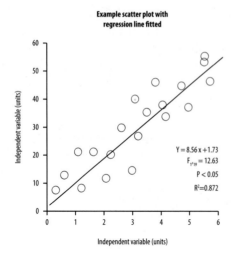

Example scatter plot with regression line fitted

$Y = 8.56x + 1.73$
$F_{1,19} = 12.63$
$P < 0.05$
$R^2 = 0.872$

predictor variables (i.e. Xs) are assessed.

Although some researchers may argue that the interchangeable use of multivariate and multivariable is simply semantics, but public health researchers believe that differentiating between the two terms is important for the field of public health. In general, models used in public health research should be described as simple or multivariable, to indicate the number of predictors, and as linear, logistic, multivariate, or proportional hazards, to indicate the type of outcome (e.g. continuous, dichotomous, repeated measures, time to event). (Bertha Hidalgo, PhD).

Summary of types of multivariate analysis

There are many different models, each with its own type of analysis:

1. Multivariate analysis of variance (MANOVA) extends the analysis of variance to cover cases where there is more than one dependent variable to be analyzed simultaneously: see also MANCOVA.

2. Multivariate regression analysis attempts to determine a formula that can describe how elements in a vector of variables respond simultaneously to changes in others. For linear relations, regression analyses here are based on forms of the general linear model.

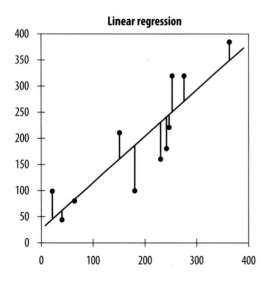

Linear regression

Fig.6.15   Models of multivariable analysis

Table 6.8   Summary of choice of statistical tests

Statistical test	Dependent variable	Independent variable
Linear regression	Quantitative	Quantitative
Multiple regression	Quantitative	Quantitative and qualitative
Logistic regression	Qualitative	Quantitative and qualitative
Linear correlation	Quantitative	Quantitative
Rank correlation	Ordinal/ranked	Ordinal/ranked

Table 6.9   2X2 table in clinical trial

Outcome	Exposure factor (intervention)		Total
	Experimental treatment	Placebo	
Yes	a	b	a+b
No	c	d	c+d
Total	a+c	b+d	a+b+c+d

3. Statistical graphics such as coordinate plots, scatterplot matrices can be used to explore multivariate data.

Statistical data analysis of clinical trials

The statistical data analysis of clinical trials consists of computing the following:

1. Odds ratio (OR)
2. Experimental event rate (EER)
3. Control event rate (CER)
4. Relative risk (RR)
5. Absolute risk reduction (ARR
6. Number needed to treat (NNT)
7. Relative risk reduction (RRR)
8. ODDS Ratio: It is the ratio between two ratios.

   OR = ad/bc

9. Experimental event rate (EER)—rate of event (risk of disease) in a group of subjects that received experimental treatment

   EER = a/a+b

10. Control event rate (CER)—rate of event (risk of disease) in group subjects that received traditional treatment or placebo.

    CER = b/b+d

11. Relative risk (RR)—is the ratio of the risk of disease in an exposed subjects group (received experiment treatment) to the rate of risk disease in a non-exposed subjects group (didn't receive experiment treatment). Relative risk indicates how more likely exposed people have an outcome than unexposed people.

RR = EER/CER

The relative risk interpretation measurement scale:

RR = 1, the intervention is an indifferent factor.

RR>1, intervention is a risk factor

RR<1, intervention is a beneficial/ protective factor

12. Absolute risk reduction (ARR) provides a way to assess the reduction in risk compared with the baseline risk and indicates how many subjects avoid the event occurrence for every 100 subjects.

    ARR = CER-EER

e.g.: In the aspirin study the EER for a cardiovascular disease (CVD) was 0.14 in the aspirin group (experimental group), and the control group event rate (CER) was 0.30. In this case ARR = 0.30 – 0.14 = 0.16

The interpretation:

The risk of CVD is 14 subjects per 100 in the group taking aspirin, and 30 in the group taking a placebo. Taking aspirin, every 16 subjects per 100 people avoid the occurrence of CVD or 160 per 1000 people, etc.

13. The number needed to treat is an added

advantage of interpreting risk data in terms of absolute risk reduction. The main meaning is to find out the number needed to treat in order to prevent one event.

NNT = 1/AAR

e.g.: in the previous example of aspirin study NNT = 1/0.16= 6.25 , then to avoid one CVD is needed to be aspirin treated 6.25 patient. This type of information helps clinicians evaluate the relative risks and benefits of a particular treatment.

14. Relative Risk Reduction (RRR) – defined as amount of risk reduction relative to the baseline

RRR = = 1 – RR

e.g.: In the previous aspirin study RRR = or 53%

The relative risk reduction tells us that, relative to the baseline risk of 30 CVD per 100 people, giving aspirin reduces the risk by 53%.

Advantages

- Give strong causality evidence
- Less bias
- Historic controls can be used in preliminary study

Disadvantages

- Expensive
- Ethical issues
- They need time
- Participant compliance

Interpretation of statistics

One of the primary purposes of statistical analysis is to provide a standardized method of presenting diverse experimental findings. This serves to facilitate the interpretation of results and to ensure a level of quality control, and deviations from these standardized procedures should be appraised critically. A failure to correct for multiple comparisons (e.g. post hoc hypothesis generation), for example, will lead to artificially low p values, as would the application of normality-dependent statistical tests to data that are not normally distributed. Nonstandard tests should always be accompanied by a brief justification and reference to avoid the perception of "test shopping" for rare or cryptic tests that may generate lower P-values. In contrast, statistical errors can also serve to undersell data, such as the failure to use a paired or one-tailed version of a t-test when appropriate, thereby reducing the statistical power.

As always, it is critical to note the difference between statistical significance and clinical significance.

There is often a temptation to distill statistics down to a single p value and apply a binary label of "significant" or "not" based on the ubiquitous 0.05 threshold. However, it is important to note that P-values themselves do not indicate the strengths of relationships, but rather the likelihoods that such relationships (as defined by the statistical test of choice) may have occurred by chance. Furthermore, true controls rarely exist in a clinical setting, and confounding variables are more often the rule than the exception. Clinically trivial results may exhibit statistical significance, and, likewise, results that fail to achieve statistical significance may nonetheless be clinically relevant.

Nevertheless, statistics are an essential component of data analysis, and a ready familiarity with this lexicon is critical to the interpretation of medical literature.

(Geoffrey C. Gurtner, M.D. Stanford University School of Medicine).

Chapter 7
PROBABILITY AND SIGNIFICANCE

Probability measures uncertainty; it lies at the heart of statistical theory. A probability measures the chance of a given event occurring.

Definition of probability

It is the chance of rejecting a true null hypothesis.

It is a positive number that lies between zero and one. If it is equal to zero, then the event *cannot* occur. If it is equal to one, then the event *must* occur.

If an event can occur in N mutually exclusive and equally likely ways, and if m of these possess a trait, E, the probability of the occurrence of E is:

$$P(E) = m/N$$

Probability introduction

Medical professionals use the term probability many times each day. For example, a physician says that a patient has a 50-50 chance of surviving a certain operation. Another physician may say that she is 95% certain that a patient has a particular disease. The clinical trials are any planned process of data collection. It consists of a number of trials (replications) under the same condition and events result in an outcome that has certain probability.

Sample space: collection of unique, non-overlapping possible outcomes of a random circumstance.

Simple event: one outcome in the sample space; a possible outcome of a random circumstance.

Event: a collection of one or more simple events in the sample space; often written as A, B, C, etc.

Complement: when the probability that an event will not happen; an event opposite to the event of interest is called a complementary event.

If A is an event, the probability of the complement is A^C or $`A$

The probability of the **complementary** event (the event *not* occurring) is one minus the probability of the event occurring. We discuss **conditional probability**, the probability of an event, given that another event has occurred.

We can calculate a probability using various approaches.

Views in probability

*   **Subjective**—Our personal degree of belief that the event will occur (e.g. that the world will come to an end in the year 2050). It is an estimate that reflects a person's opinion, or best guess about whether an outcome will occur.

    This is important in medicine because it forms the basis of a physician's opinion (based on information gained in the history and physical examination) about whether a patient has a specific disease. Such estimates can be changed with the results of diagnostic procedures.

- **Frequentist**—the proportion of times the event would occur if we were to repeat the experiment a large number of times (e.g. the number of times we would get a 'head' if we tossed a fair coin 1,000 times).

- *A priori*—this requires knowledge of the theoretical *model*, called the **probability distribution**, which describes the probabilities of all possible outcomes of the 'experiment'. For example, genetic theory allows us to describe the probability distribution for eye colour in a baby born to a blue-eyed woman and brown-eyed man by initially specifying all possible genotypes of eye colour in the baby and their probabilities.

Objectives in probability

Classical example

It is well known that the probability of flipping a fair coin and getting a "tail" is 0.50.

If a coin is flipped 10 times, is there a guarantee, that exactly five tails will be observed?

What it the coin is flipped 100 times? With 1,000 flips?

As the number of flips becomes larger, the proportion of coin flips that result in tails approaches 0.50.

Relative frequency

Assuming that an experiment can be repeated many times and assuming that there are one or more outcomes that can result from each repetition; then, the probability of a given outcome is the number of times that outcome occurs divided by the total number of repetitions.

Marginal probabilities

They are called marginal probabilities because they appear on the margins of a probability table. It is probability of a single outcome.

Conditional probabilities

It is the probability of an event on condition that certain criteria is satisfied.

Example

If 20 subjects were selected randomly what is the probability that one has a blood group O?

Here the total possible outcomes constitute a subset (females) of 20 out of the total number of 100 subjects.

This probability is termed as probability of O given F.

$P(O\backslash F) = 20/50$

$= 0.40$

Joint probability

It is the probability of occurrence of two or more events together.

Example

Probability of being male and belong to the blood group AB. Five males had blood group AB out of 100 subjects. The probability is as follows:

$P(M \text{ and } AB) = P(M \cap AB)$

$= 5/100$

$= 0.05$

$\cap$ = intersection

The rules of probability

We can use the rules of probability to add and multiply probabilities.

- **The addition rule**—if two events, A and B, are *mutually exclusive* (i.e. each event precludes the other), then the probability that either one or the other occurs is equal to the sum of their probabilities. E.g., if the probabilities that an adult patient in a particular dental practice has no missing teeth, some missing teeth or is edentulous (i.e. has no teeth) are 0.67, 0.24 and 0.09, respectively, then the probability that a patient has some teeth is $0.67 + 0.24 = 0.91$.

- **The multiplication rule**—if two events, A and B, are *independent* (i.e. the occurrence of one event is not contingent on the other), then the probability that both events occur is equal to the product of the probability of each:

Prob (A *and* B) = Prob (A) Prob (B)

e.g. if two unrelated patients are waiting in the dentist's surgery, the probability that both of them have no missing teeth is 0.67—0.67 = 0.45.

Probability distributions: The theory

A **random variable** is a quantity that can take any one of a set of mutually exclusive values with a given probability. A **probability distribution** shows the probabilities of all possible values of the random variable. It is a theoretical distribution that is expressed mathematically, and has a mean and variance that are analogous to those of an empirical distribution. Each probability distribution is defined by certain **parameters** which are summary measures (e.g. mean, variance) characterizing that distribution (i.e. knowledge of them allows the distribution to be fully described). These parameters are estimated in the sample by relevant **statistics**. Depending on whether the random variable is discrete or continuous, the probability distribution can be either discrete or continuous.

- **Discrete** (e.g. Binomial, Poisson)—we can derive probabilities corresponding to every possible value of the random variable. *The sum of all such probabilities is one*.

- **Continuous** (e.g. normal, Chi-squared, *t*

and *F*)—we can only derive the probability of the random variable, *x*, taking values in certain ranges (because there are infinitely many values of *x*). If the horizontal axis represents the values of *x*, we can draw a curve from the equation of the distribution (the **probability density function**); it resembles an empirical relative frequency distribution.

The total area under the curve is one; this area represents the probability of all possible events. The probability that *x* lies between two limits is equal to the area under the curve between these values. For convenience, tables have been produced to enable us to evaluate probabilities of interest for commonly used continuous probability distributions. These are particularly useful in the context of confidence intervals and hypothesis testing.

One of the most important distributions in statistics is the **Normal distribution**. Its probability density function is:

1. Completely described by two parameters, the *mean* (m) and the *variance* (S^2);
2. Bell-shaped (unimodal)
3. Symmetrical about its mean
4. Shifted to the right if the mean is increased and to the left if the mean is decreased (assuming constant variance)
5. Flattened as the variance is increased but becomes more peaked as the variance is decreased (for a fixed mean)

Additional properties are that:

1. The mean and median of a normal distribution are equal
2. The probability that a normally distributed random variable, *x*, with mean, m, and standard deviation, s, lies between:

These intervals may be used to define **reference intervals.**

The standard normal distribution

There are infinitely many normal distributions depending on the values of m and s.

• The Standard Normal distribution has a **mean of zero** and a **variance of one**.

• If the random variable, x, has a normal distribution with mean, m, and variance, S2, then the **Standardized Normal Deviate (SND)**, is a random variable that has a Standard Normal Distribution.

Discrete probability distributions

The random variable that defines the probability distribution is discrete.

The sum of the probabilities of all possible mutually exclusive events is one.

The Binomial distribution

• Suppose, in a given situation, there are only two outcomes, 'success' and 'failure'. For example, we may be interested in whether a woman conceives (a success) or does not conceive (a failure) after *in vitro* fertilization (IVF). If we look at $n = 100$ unrelated women undergoing IVF (each with the same probability of conceiving), the binomial random variable is the observed number of conceptions (successes). Often this concept is explained in terms of n independent repetitions of a trial (e.g. 100 tosses of a coin) in which the outcome is either success (e.g. head) or failure.

• The two parameters that describe the Binomial distribution are n, the number of individuals in the sample (or repetitions of a trial) and p, the true probability of success for each individual (or in each trial).

• Its **mean** (the value for the random variable that we *expect* if we look at n individuals, or repeat the trial n times) is np. Its **variance** is np(1 - p). When n is small, the distribution is skewed to the right if p < 0.5, and to the left if p > 0.5. The distribution becomes more symmetrical as the sample size increases (Fig. 8.4) and approximates the Normal distribution if both np and n(1 - p) are greater than 5.

• We can use the properties of the Binomial distribution when making inferences about **proportions**. In particular, we often use the Normal approximation to the Binomial distribution when analysing proportions.

The Poisson distribution

The Poisson random variable is the **count** of the number of events that occur independently and randomly in time or space at some average rate, m. For example, the number of hospital admissions per day typically follows the Poisson distribution. We can use our knowledge of the Poisson distribution to calculate the probability of a certain number of admissions on any particular day.

1. The parameter that describes the Poisson distribution is the **mean**, i.e. the average rate, m.

2. The **mean** equals the **variance** in the Poisson distribution.

3. It is a right skewed distribution if the mean is small, but becomes more symmetrical as the mean increases, when it approximates a normal distribution.

Statistical significance based on probability

The probability that the statistical association found between the variables is due to random chance.

The preset probability is set sufficiently low that one would act on the result; frequently p = 0.01 or 0.05.

The multivariable analysis like linear

regression, logistic regression are based on probability models.

When statistical tests result in a probability less than the preset limit the results are said to be statistically significant, i.e. $p < 0.05$.

Examples

1. If tuberculous meningitis had a case fatality of 20%:

   a. Find the probability that this disease would be fatal in two randomly selected patients (the two events are independent).

   b. If two patients are selected randomly what is the probability that at least one of them will die?

   c. P (first die and second die) = 20% + 20% = 40% = 0.4

   d. P (first die or second die)

   e. = P (first die) + P (second die) - P (both die)

      = 20% + 20% - 4%

      = 36%

2. In a normally distributed population, the probability that a subject's blood cholesterol level will be lower than 1 SD below the mean is 16% and the probability of being blood cholesterol level higher than 2 SD above the mean is 2.5%. What is the probability that a randomly selected subject will have a blood cholesterol level lower than 1 SD below the mean or higher than 2 SD above the mean?

   P (blood cholesterol level < 1 SD below the mean or 2 SD above the mean) = 16% +2.5%

   = 18.5%

Chapter 8

SAMPLE SIZE CALCULATIONS

THE IMPORTANCE OF SAMPLE SIZE

If the number of patients in our study is small, we may have inadequate power to detect an important existing effect, and we shall have wasted all our resources. On the other hand, if the sample size is unduly large, the study may be unnecessarily time consuming, expensive and unethical, depriving some of the patients of the superior treatment. We therefore have to choose the optimal sample size which strikes a balance between the implications of making a Type I or Type II error. Unfortunately, in order to calculate the sample size required, we have to have some idea of the results we expect in the study.

SAMPLE SIZE CALCULATIONS IN MEDICAL RESEARCH

Sample size contributes to the statistical precision of the estimate.

Increasing the sample size decreases the probability of type I and type II error.

Epi info software determines sample size. Raosoft can also be used.

First, the investigator must specify a value for alpha, the likelihood that the null hypothesis (of no difference) will be rejected when it is in fact true.

Although alpha can be chosen as any value between 0 and 1, by convention it is usually taken to be 0.05 based on a two-tailed test of statistical significance.

Smaller values of alpha will require larger sample sizes. Specifying a one tailed test will result in a smaller required sample size, but should be rarely done because it requires that the direction of an association be known with complete certainty.

Second, the investigator must specify a value for beta, the likelihood that the null hypothesis is not rejected (i.e. an observed difference is declared to be "not significant" when the null hypothesis, in fact, is not true. Beta is usually set at 0.10 or 0.20. The power of a statistical test is 1 - beta. Thus, with beta equal to 0.10, the power to reject the null hypothesis when it is not true is 1 - 0.10 or 0.90. The smaller the value of beta, the greater the power, and the larger the sample size that is needed.

Third, the investigator must specify the size of the effect the study is desired to detect. For cohort or experimental studies with outcome measures defined as yes/no, the effect could be either a difference in relative risk or a difference in outcome rates. The effect measure is usually an odds ratio for case-control studies. The smaller the effect size to be detected, the larger the sample size that will be needed.

Finally, the investigator must provide an estimate of the variance in measures of exposure and/or outcome. For cohort and experimental studies, if the outcome of interest is a yes/no variable, the investigator must specify the proportion of the unexposed population expected to develop the condition of interest because the variance depends on this proportion. Rare outcomes require larger sample size. In case-control studies, the investigator must specify the expected proportion of exposed controls. Rare exposures require larger samples sizes in case-control studies. In studies with continuously distributed variables either as exposures or as outcomes (e.g. blood pressure), the required sample size is dependent on the variance of the measure, which must be specified by the investigator. The greater the variance, the larger the sample size that is needed to detect an association of a given size.

Sample-size estimation for more complex study designs may require the investigator to specify other quantities. For example, to estimate the appropriate sample size for a study that involves randomization of units (e.g. communities, physician practices), it is necessary to specify the expected correlation of measures within individuals in the randomized unit. Estimation of sample size for survival differences in a follow-up study requires specification of the expected rate of loss-to-follow-up and the expected change over time in the rate of disease.

Requirements

We shall explain how to calculate the optimal sample size in simple situations; often more complex designs can be simplified for the purpose of calculating the sample size. If our investigation involves a number of tests, we concentrate on the most important or evaluate the sample size required for each and choose the largest.

Our focus is the calculation of the optimal sample size in relation to a proposed hypothesis test. However, it is possible to base the sample size calculation on other aspects of the study, such as on the precision of an estimate or on the width of a confidence interval (the process

usually adopted in equivalence and non-inferiority studies).

To calculate the optimal sample size for a test, we need to specify the following quantities *at the design stage of the investigation*.

- **Power**—The chance of detecting, as statistically significant, a specified effect if it exits. We usually choose a power of at least 80%.

- **Significance level**—The cut-off level below which we will reject the null hypothesis, i.e. it is the maximum probability of incorrectly concluding that there is an effect. We usually fix this as 0.05 or, occasionally, as 0.01, and reject the null hypothesis if the *P*-value is less than this value.

- **Variability** of the observations e.g. the standard deviation, if we have a numerical variable or proportion if we have a catagorical variables.

- **Smallest effect of interest**—The magnitude of the effect that is clinically important and which we do not want to overlook. This is often a *difference* (e.g. difference in means or proportions). Sometimes it is expressed as a multiple of the standard deviation of the observations (the **standardized difference**).

It is relatively simple to choose the power and significance level of the test that suit the requirements of our study. The choice is usually governed by the implications of a Type I and a Type II error, but may be specified by the regulatory bodies in some drug licensing studies. Given a particular clinical scenario, it is possible to specify the effect we regard as clinically important. The real difficulty lies in providing an estimate of the variation in a numerical variable before we have collected the data. We may be able to obtain this information from other published studies with similar outcomes or we may need to carry out a **pilot study**.

Methodology

We can calculate sample size in a number of ways, each of which requires essentially the same information.

General formulae—these can be complex but may be necessary in some situations {e.g. to retain power in a cluster randomized trial, we multiply the sample size that would be required if we were carrying out individual randomization by the design effect equal to [1 + (*m* - 1) r], where *m* is the average cluster size and r is the intraclass correlation coefficient.

Quick formulae—These exist for particular power values and significance levels for some hypothesis tests (e.g. Lehr's formulae).

- **Special tables**[1]—These exist for different situations (e.g. for *t*-tests, Chi-squared tests, test of the correlation coefficient, comparing two survival curves and for equivalence studies).

- **Altman's nomogram**—This is an easy to use diagram which is appropriate for various tests. Details are given in the next section.

- **Computer software**—This has the advantage that results can be presented graphically or in tables to show the effect of changing the factors (e.g. power, size of effect) on the required sample size.

Altman's nomogram

Notation

The notation for using Altman's nomogram to estimate the sample size of two *equally sized* groups of observations for three frequently used hypothesis tests of means and proportions.

Method

For each test, we calculate the standardized difference and join its value on the left hand axis of the nomogram to the power we have specified on the right hand vertical axis. The

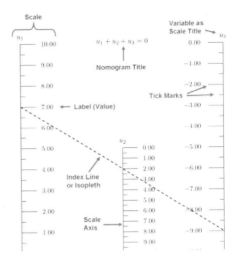

Fig.8.1   Models of multivariable analysis

required sample size is indicated at the point at which the resulting line and sample size axis meet.

Note that we can also use the nomogram to evaluate the power of a hypothesis test for a given sample size. Occasionally, this is useful if we wish to know, retrospectively, whether we can attribute lack of significance in a hypothesis test to an inadequately sized sample.

Remember, also, that a wide confidence interval for the effect of interest indicates low power.

Quick formulae

For the unpaired *t*-test and Chi-squared test, we can use **Lehr's formula** for calculating the sample size for a power of 80% and a two-sided significance level of 0.05. The required sample size in each group is:

If the standardized difference is small, this formula overestimates the sample size. Note that a numerator of 21 (instead of 16) relates to a power of 90%.

Power statement

It is often essential and always useful to include a power statement in a study protocol or in the methods section of a paper. CONSORT statement to show that careful thought has been given to sample size at the design stage of the investigation.

A typical statement might be 84 patients in each group were required for the unpaired *t*-test to have a 90% chance of detecting a difference in means of 2.5 days (SD = five days) at the 5% level of significance.

Adjustments

We may wish to adjust the sample size:

- to allow for **losses to follow-up** by recruiting more patients into the study at the outset. If we believe that the drop-out rate will be $r\%$, then the adjusted sample size is obtained by multiplying the unadjusted sample size by $100/(100 - r)$;

- to have independent **groups of different sizes**. This may be desirable when one group is restricted in size, perhaps because the disease is rare in a case-control study or because the novel drug treatment is in short supply. Note, however, that the imbalance in numbers usually results in a larger overall sample size when compared to a balanced design if a similar level of power is to be maintained. If the ratio of the sample sizes in the two groups is k (e.g. $k = 3$ if we require one group to be three times the size of the other), the adjusted overall sample size is where N is the unadjusted overall sample size calculated for equally sized groups. Then $N¢/(1 + k)$ of these patients will be in the smaller group and the remaining patients will be in the larger group.

Single mean

Standard Deviation ^{2} ÷ Standard Error ^{2}

We wish to determine the mean birth weight of the infants. The mean weight is expected to be 3000 G ± SD 500. Standard error will be 25 G.

$500^2 ÷ 25^2 = 250,000 ÷ 625 = 400$ **Infants**

Single rate

Rate ÷ Standard Error ^{2}

The maternal mortality in the country is expected to be 70 per

10,000 live births. The permissible SE is 5 /10,000.

(70/ 10,000) ÷ 5/10,000 = 28,000 live births

Single proportion

Proportion – (100 – Proportion) ÷ Standard Error ^{2}

Difference between two means

(SD1 2 + SD2 2) ÷ Standard Error ^{2}

Difference between two rates

(Rate1 + Rate2) ÷ Standard Error ^{2}

Sample size for surveys

Sample Size = Confidence Limits ^{2} Proportion without disease

Margin of Error ^{2} Proportion with disease

Prevalence 5 % Confidence Limit 95 % Margin of Error 7 %

$$1.96\ 2 \times 0.95\ (1 - 0.05)$$
$$0.7\ 2 \qquad 0.05$$
$$784\ x \qquad 19 = 14,896$$

SAMPLE SIZE CALCULATIONS FOR TWO GROUPS

The sample size calculations for two groups are dependent on different study designs.

The sample size for any study depends on:

1. Acceptable level of significance
2. Power of the study
3. Expected effect size
4. Underlying event rate in population
5. Standard deviation in population
6. Allowable error

1. $n = \dfrac{2(Z_\alpha + Z_{1\,\beta})}{\Delta^2}$

2. $n = \left[\dfrac{Z\alpha S^{1-2}}{E}\right]$

n   = required sample size

σ =   standard deviation

Δ =   difference in effect of two interventions

Z_α =   Z is constant. It is set by convention according to the accepted α error.

$Z_{1-\beta}$ =   Z is constant. It is set by convention according to the accepted power of study.

S   =   Standard deviation

E   =   Allowable error

3. Fleiss' formula for sample size:

$$n = \dfrac{[Z_{\alpha 2}\,(r+1)pq + Z_{1}{-}_{\beta}\sqrt{rp_1q_1 + p_2q_2}]}{r(p_1 - p_2)^2}$$

4. $n = \dfrac{Z^2 pq}{d^2}$

where

Z   = 1.96 for confidence level 95%

p   = prevalence

q   = 1 – prevalence

d   = margin of cross (usually 0.05)

p_1 = prevalence in group 1

p_2 = Prevalence in group 2

SAMPLE SIZE CALCULATIONS IN EXPERIMENTAL STUDIES

The sample size is the number of patients or other experimental units included in a study, and one of the first practical steps in designing a trial is the choice of the sample size needed to answer the research question. Also in the critical appraisal of the results of published trials, evaluating the sample size required to answer the research question is an important step in interpreting the relevance of these results. It is therefore not surprising that one of the most frequent requests that statistical consultants get from investigators are sample size calculations or sample size justifications.

Techniques for sample size calculations are described in most conventional statistical textbooks. However, the wide range of formulas that can be used for specific situations and study designs makes it difficult for most investigators to decide which method to use. Moreover, these calculations are sensitive to errors because small differences in selected parameters can lead to large differences in the sample size.

The main aim of a sample size calculation is to determine the number of participants needed to detect a clinically relevant treatment effect. Pre-study calculation of the required sample size is warranted in the majority of quantitative studies. Usually, the number of patients in a study is restricted because of ethical, cost and time considerations. However, if the sample size is too small, one may not be able to detect an important existing effect, whereas samples that are too large may waste time, resources and money. It is therefore important to optimize the sample size. Moreover, calculating the sample size in the design stage of the study is increasingly becoming a requirement when seeking ethical committee approval for a research project.

COMPONENTS OF SAMPLE SIZE CALCULATIONS

In order to calculate the sample size, it is required to have some idea of the results expected in a study. In general, the greater the variability in the outcome variable, the larger the sample size required to assess whether an observed effect is a true effect. On the other hand, the more effective (or harmful!) a tested treatment is, the smaller the sample size needed to detect this positive or negative effect. Calculating the sample size for a trial requires four basic components:

The type I error (alpha). Clinical studies are usually performed in a sample from a population rather than in the whole study population. In research, we are testing hypotheses to determine whether (results in) particular samples differ from each other. On the one hand, the null hypothesis (H_0) hypothesizes that the groups of subjects (samples) that are being compared are not different, that is they come from the same source population. The alternative hypothesis (H_1), on the other hand, hypothesizes that these groups are different and that therefore they seem to be drawn from different source populations. Sample size calculations are needed to define at what number of subjects it becomes quite unlikely that adding more subjects will change the conclusion.

In the process of hypothesis–testing, two fundamental errors can occur. These errors are called type I and type II errors.

The type I error (alpha) measures the probability that, given the H_0 that the samples come from the same source population, the differences found are likely to happen. In other words, the alpha represents the chance of a falsely rejecting H_0 and picking up a false-positive effect. The alpha is most commonly fixed at 0.05, which means that the researcher desires a <5% chance of drawing a false-positive conclusion.

Instead of a false-positive conclusion, investigators can also draw a false-negative conclusion. In such cases, they conclude that there is no difference between two groups or treatments when in reality there is, or in other words, they falsely accept the H_0 that the compared samples come from the same source population. This is called a type II error (beta).

Conventionally, the beta is set at a level of 0.20, meaning that the researcher desires a <20% chance of a false-negative conclusion.

For the calculation of the sample size, one needs to know the power of a study. The power reflects the ability to pick up an effect that is present in a population using a test based on a sample from that population (true positive). The power is the complement of beta: 1-beta. So, in case of a beta of 0.20, the power would be 0.80 or 80%, representing the probability of avoiding a false-negative conclusion, or the chance of correctly rejecting a null hypothesis.

The smallest effect of interest

The smallest effect of interest is the minimal difference between the studied groups that the investigator wishes to detect and is often referred to as the minimal clinically relevant difference, sometimes abbreviated as MCRD. This should be a difference that the investigator believes to be clinically relevant and biologically plausible. For continuous outcome variables, the minimal clinically relevant difference is a numerical difference. For example, if body weight is the outcome of a trial, an investigator could choose a difference of 5 kg as the minimal clinically relevant difference. In a trial with a binary outcome, for example the effect of a drug on the development of a myocardial infarction (yes/no), an investigator should estimate a relevant difference between the event rates in both treatment groups and could choose, for instance, a difference of 10% between the treatment group and the control group as minimal clinically relevant difference. Even a small change in the expected difference with treatment has a major effect on the estimated sample size, as the sample size is inversely proportional to the square of the difference. For instance, if one would need 1,000 subjects to detect an absolute difference of 4.8%, 4,000 subjects per treatment group would be required to detect a 2.4% difference.

The variability

Finally, the sample size calculation is based on using the population variance of a given outcome variable that is estimated by means of the standard deviation (SD) in case of a continuous outcome. Because the variance is usually an unknown quantity, investigators often use an estimate obtained from a pilot study or use information from a previously performed study. For example, in an echocardiography substudy of the Australian Initiating Dialysis Early And Late (IDEAL) Study, Cooper *et al.* aim to determine whether the timing of dialysis initiation has an effect on left ventricular mass. For their sample size calculation, the investigators used recent data from another laboratory indicating that the mean left ventricular mass in renal failure patients in Australia is 140 g/m² with an SD of 60 g/m².

Sometimes, the minimal clinically relevant difference and the variability are combined and expressed as a multiple of the SD of the observations; the standardized difference. The standardized difference is also referred to as the effect size and can be calculated as:

A summary of all components of sample size calculations is presented in Table two.

HOW TO CALCULATE THE SAMPLE SIZE FOR RANDOMIZED CONTROLLED TRIALS

Formulas for sample size calculation differ depending on the type of study design and the studies outcome(s). These calculations are particularly of interest in the design of randomized controlled trials (RCTs). In RCTs, a lot of money is invested, and it is therefore important to be sufficiently sure that enough patients are included in the study arms in order to find as statistically significant a difference that we assume there is in the population. In general, sample size calculations are performed based on the primary outcome of the study.

Based on two examples, we will now demonstrate how to calculate sample size using the simplest formulas for an RCT comparing two groups of equal size. Suppose one wished

to study the effect of a new hypertensive drug on (i) systolic blood pressure (SBP) as a continuous outcome and (ii) SBP as a binary outcome, i.e. below or above 140 mmHg (hypertension yes/no).

SBP as a continuous outcome

Simplest formula for a continuous outcome and equal sample sizes in both groups, assuming: alpha = 0.05 and power = 0.80 (beta = 0.20).

n = the sample size in each of the groups

μ_1 = population mean in treatment Group 1

μ_2 = population mean in treatment Group 2

$\mu_1 - \mu_2$ = the difference the investigator wishes to detect

σ^2 = population variance (SD)

a = conventional multiplier for alpha = 0.05

b = conventional multiplier for power = 0.80

When the significance level alpha is chosen at 0.05, like in these examples, one should enter the value 1.96 for a in the formula. Similarly, when beta is chosen at 0.20, the value 0.842 should be filled in for b in the formula. These multipliers for conventional values of alpha and beta can be performed.

Suppose the investigators consider a difference in SBP of 15 mmHg between the treated and the control group $(\mu_1 - \mu_2)$ as clinically relevant and specified such an effect to be detected with 80% power (0.80) and a significance level alpha of 0.05. Past experience with similar experiments, with similar measuring methods and similar subjects, suggests that the data will be approximately normally distributed with an SD of 20 mmHg. Now we have all of the specifications needed for determining sample size using the approach. Entering the values in the formula yields: $2 \times [(1.96 + 0.842)^2 \times 20^2] / 15^2 = 27.9$, this means that a sample size of 28 subjects per group is needed to answer the research question.

SBP as a binary outcome

For a study with a binary outcome, calculating the required sample size is slightly more complicated. It should be calculated based on the number of events rather than on the number of people in the study. The number of events can be increased either by choosing higher risk patients, by increasing the follow-up time, or by increasing the sample size.

Simplest formula for a binary outcome and equal sample sizes in both groups, assuming: alpha = 0.05 and power = 0.80 (beta = 0.20).

n = the sample size in each of the groups

p_1 = proportion of subjects with hypertension in treatment Group 1

q_1 = proportion of subjects without hypertension in treatment Group 1 (= $1 - p_1$)

p_2 = proportion of subjects with hypertension in treatment Group 2

q_2 = proportion of subjects without hypertension in treatment Group 2 (= $1 - p_2$)

x = the difference the investigator wishes to detect

a = conventional multiplier for alpha = 0.05

b = conventional multiplier for power = 0.80

In this case, we suppose that the investigators consider a difference in event rate of 10% (0.10) as clinically relevant. Based on recently published findings from studies with a similar design, they expect that the proportion of subjects with hypertension in the treated group will be ~20% (p_1 = 0.20) and in the control group, ~30% (p_2 = 0.30). This automatically means that q_1 and q_2 are 0.80 and 0.70, respectively. Again, the investigators assume a power of 80% (0.80) and an alpha of 0.05, which means that the value 1.96 should be filled in for a and the value 0.842 should be

filled in for b. We can now enter all values in the formula presented in Box 2: $[(1.96 + 0.842)^2 \times (0.20 \times 0.80 + 0.30 \times 0.70)] / 0.10^2 = 290.5$, this means that a sample size of 291 subjects per group is needed to answer the research question.

Many of the formulas to calculate sample size are not straightforward. For some simple clinical trials, nomograms or graphs can be used to estimate the sample size required for the study. An example of such a nomogram is published by Altman. However, one should keep in mind that, although these graphical methods work well, they often make assumptions about the type of data and statistical tests to be used.

Other outcome types

In many trials, the outcomes may not be continuous or binary as above, but instead may be survival (e.g. time to event). In these cases, the details of calculation differ, but using the four aforementioned components, persist through calculations with other types of outcomes. However, other assumptions can be necessary.

Other study designs than RCTs

Although the calculation of sample size is based on the same principles for all parallel study designs, the formulas for sample size calculations for other study designs than RCTs often need some adaptations. For example, published formulas for case-control designs provide sample sizes required to determine that an odds ratio is significantly different from one, after adjustment for potential confounders. Also, sample size calculations for special types of RCTs, like cluster-randomized trials, in which health interventions are allocated randomly to intact clusters, communities, health centres or practices rather than to individual subjects, need an alternative approach. The same holds true for trials with a crossover design, because these studies compare the results of two treatments on the same group of patients. The sample size calculated for a crossover study can also be used for a study that compares the value of a variable after treatment with its value before treatment. Finally, sample size calculations for clinical trials testing the equivalence rather than the superiority between two treatments need another approach. These equivalence or non-inferiority trials usually demand higher sample sizes. The aforementioned alternative calculations are less common and more complicated and will in most cases require statistical assistance.

Common pitfalls

The calculation of the sample size is troubled by a large amount of imprecision, because investigators rarely have good estimates of the parameters necessary for the calculation. Unfortunately, the required sample size is very sensitive to the choice of these parameters.

The effects of selecting alpha and the power

In most cases, the conventional choices of an alpha of 0.05 and a power of 0.80 are adequate. However, dependent on the topic studied, other assumptions can be made. Different assumptions of alpha and the power will directly influence the sample size. A lower alpha and a higher power will both lead to a larger sample size and as a result to higher costs. To be aware of the influence of changes in these parameters, it can be helpful to perform sample size calculations for different values of the parameters (sensitivity analyses). In case of doubt, one should generally choose the largest sample size.

Estimating the difference and SD

Studies often aim to determine parameters like event rates in the treated group and the control group. Needing to estimate these parameters before the start of the study therefore seems strange for many investigators. It is, however, important to realize that the parameters they are estimating in order to calculate the required sample size are not the population parameters as such, but the treatment effects they consider biologically plausible and clinically relevant.

In most studies, investigators estimate the difference of interest and the standard deviation based on results from a pilot study, published data or on their own knowledge and opinion. This means that the calculation of an appropriate sample size partly relies on subjective choices or crude estimates of certain factors which may seem rather artificial to some. Unless the pilot study was large, using information from a pilot study often results in unreliable estimates of the variability and the minimal clinically relevant difference. By definition, pilot studies are underpowered, and the observed difference in a pilot study is therefore an imprecise estimate of the difference in the population. Not accounting for this sampling error will lead to underpowered studies. Also published reports could provide an estimate of the outcome in the control group. Although they often incorporate a lot of differences with the study one aims to perform, such as dissimilar eligibility criteria, endpoints and treatments, some information on the control group usually exists. Finally, another approach is to survey experts in the field to determine what difference would need to be demonstrated for them to adapt a new treatment in terms of costs and risks.

After mentioning these pitfalls, it may seem useless to perform a sample size calculation. However, even if based on estimates and assumptions, a sample size calculation is considerably more useful than a completely arbitrary choice.

Post hoc sample calculations

Sometimes, published studies wrongfully report their 'power' instead of 95% confidence intervals (CIs). The power should always be calculated prior to a study to determine the required sample size, since it is the pre-study probability that the study will detect a minimum effect regarded as clinically significant. After the study is conducted, one should not perform any 'post hoc' power calculations. Once the effect of the study is known, investigators should use the 95% CI to express the amount of uncertainty around the effect estimate.

Reporting of sample size calculations

According to the CONSORT statement, sample size calculations should be reported and justified in all published RCTs. These calculations provide important information. Firstly, they specify the primary endpoint, which safeguards against changing the planned outcome and claiming a large effect on an outcome which was not the original primary outcome. Secondly, knowing the planned size alerts readers to potential problems, like problems with the recruitment or an early stop of the trial. Readers of a published trial should be able to find all assumptions underlying the sample size calculation; the alpha, the power, the event rate in the control group and the treatment effect of interest (or the event rate in the treated group). Many studies only include statements like 'we calculated that the sample size in each treatment group should be 250 at an alpha of 0.05 and a power of 0.80'. However, such a statement is almost meaningless because it neglects the estimates for the effect of interest and the variability. Based on an example from the IDEAL Study, we can illustrate that a better way to report these calculations would be: 'A clinically significant effect of 10% or more over the three years would be of interest. Assuming 3-year survival rates in the control group and the intervention group of 64% and 74% respectively, with a two-sided significance of 0.05 and a power of 0.8, a total of 800–1000 patients will be required.

Although, ideally, all four components conventionally required for sample size calculation should be published, Charles *et al.* recently showed that of 215 published reports of RCTs, 10 (5%) did not report any sample size calculation, and 92 (43%) did not report all the required parameters. Moreover, a Danish study by *Chan et al.* demonstrated that, also in study protocols, sample size calculations are often poorly reported, and that explicit discrepancies between protocols and published papers are common. They found that only 11 of 62 (18%) identified studies described existing sample size calculations fully and consistently in both the protocol and the publication.

Chapter 9

REFERENCE WRITING

References are presented in medical writing style. Most common is the vancouver style in medical literature; however, some medical journals prefer the APA Reference writing style.

APA reference writing

1. Book

Morales, L. (1987). The history of Cuba. New York: Franklin Watts.

Ellington, W., Jr., & Henrickson, E.B. (1995). The elements of dance (3rd ed.). New York: Macmillan.

Oregon State University Soil Ecology Center (1982). A directory of Community Supported Agriculture (CSA) Farms. Columbus, OH: Natural Resources Institute.

2. Book chapter

Tizol, W.P. (1976). Brain function and memory. In J.M.O. Corney & H.L. Center (Eds.), An inside look at what we think we know. (pp. 154-184). Springfield, IL: American Psychiatric Press.

3. Journal article

Bauzá, R.H. (1982). Manitoba nematodes. Journal of Cool Nematodes, 10, 252-264.

Gillespie, R.C., & Tupac, R.M. (1976). How confident people dance. American Dancing, 225, 82-90.

The lamb business. (11 Sept. 1992). Willamette Valley Lamb, 97, 47-48.

4. Magazine article

Pozo, E. R. (19 Nov. 2008). The way she loved me. Personal Literature, 290, 1113-1120.

5. Encyclopedia article

Parker, S.A. (1947). Fetal development. In International encyclopedia of pregnancy (Vol. 7, pp. 202-207). New York: Aesculapius Publishers.

6. Newspaper article

Amazing women. (12 Jan. 1955). The Journal News, pp. D11, D14.

7. Electronic journal article from a database

Tjader, J.W., Coltrane, J.A., & Taylor, A.A. (1995). A history of mockery. American Psychologist, 50, 750-765. Retrieved from PsycINFO database.

8. Electronic journal article (print version)

Rodriguez, G., Puente, S., & Mayfield , J. (2001). Role of upbringing in family attitudes. [Electronic version]. Journal of Family Research, 5, 117-123.

9. Website

Summers, M. (2007) Cool scenes. Retrieved August 27, 2007.

Vancouver research writing

When writing a reference list in the Vancouver style, it is required to remember the following:

Arrange your list chronologically.

- Number all references.
- List the first six authors followed by 'et al.' if there are more than six authors.
- Use official abbreviations for titles of journals (if available).

Citations within the text of your paper are identified with a number in round brackets.

Example: Jones (8) has argued that…

- References are numbered consecutively in the order they are first used in the text. The full citations will be included in the Reference List at the end of your document, with matching numbers identifying each reference.
- When multiple references are cited together, use a hyphen to indicate a series of inclusive numbers. Use commas to indicate a series of non-inclusive numbers. A citation with these references (4, 5, 6, 7, 14, 19) is abbreviated to (4-7, 14, 19).

  Example: Multiple clinical trials (4-6, 9) show…
- The original number used for a reference is reused each time the reference is cited.

  Example: "…the theory was first put forward by Lee (7) in 1999, but there was disagreement (3, 5, 8) over its importance."
- Include the page number for any direct quotes or specific ideas.

  Example: "…has been proven demonstrably false." (4, p23)
- The citation in brackets is placed after

any commas and periods, and before any colons and semi-colons.

Example: …a new definition. (13, p111-2)…this option is preferred (11);

Indirect citations

An indirect source is when one author is quoted in the text of another author. These types of citations are generally not accepted in Vancouver Style, so seek permission from your instructor. Include the author and date of the original source in the text. Use "as cited in" or "as discussed in" to say where you found the quotation and provide the citation to that reference.

Example: James Wallace (2001) argued (cited by 5, p26), that…

Reference list

Provide full citations in your Reference List, included starting as a **new page** at the end of your document. Follow the examples included in this guide for different types of resources:

- Books
- Articles in Journals
- Websites
- Other Resources
- Personal Communication

Multiple authors

Cite authors in the same way for all types of resources:

articles, websites, videos, etc.

List up to the first **six** authors/editors, and use "et al." for any additional authors.

1. Books

Standard format for books

Author surname initials. Title: subtitle. Edition (if not the first). Place of publication:

Date of publication.

Book with one author or editor

1. Mason J., Concepts In Dental Public Health. Philadelphia: Lippincott Williams & Wilkins; 2005.
2. Ireland R, editor. Clinical Textbook of Dental Hygiene and Therapy. Oxford: Blackwell Munksgaard; 2006.

Two–six authors/editors

1. Miles DA, Van Dis ML, Williamson GF, Jensen CW.
   Radiographic imaging for the dental team. 4th ed. St. Louis: Saunders Elsevier; 2009.
2. Dionne RA, Phero JC, Becker DE, editors. Management of pain and anxiety in the dental office. Philadelphia: WB Saunders; 2002.

More than six authors/editors

Fauci AS, Braunwald E, Kasper DL, Hauser SL, Longo DL,

Jameson JL, et al., editors. Harrison's Principles of Internal Medicine. 17th ed. New York: McGraw Hill; 2008.

Organization as author

Canadian Dental Hygienists Association. Dental Hygiene: definition and scope. Ottawa:

Canadian Dental Hygienists Association; 1995.

No Author/editor

Scott's Canadian Dental Directory 2008. 9th ed. Toronto: Scott's Directories; 2007.

Government Document

Canada. Environmental Health Directorate. Radiation Protection in Dentistry: recommended safety procedures for the use of dental x-ray equipment. Safety Code 30. Ottawa: Ministry of Health; 2000.

Chapter in a book

Alexander RG. Considerations in creating a beautiful smile. In: Romano R, editor. The Art of the Smile. London: Quintessence Publishing; 2005. p. 187-210.

e-book

Irfan A., Protocols For Predictable Aesthetic Dental Restorations [Internet]. Oxford: Blackwell Munksgaard; 2006 [cited 2009 May 21]. Available from Netlibrary:

http://cclsw2.vcc.ca:2048/login?url=http://www.netLibrary.com/urlapi.asp?action=summary&v=1&bookid=181691

2. Articles in journals

Journal articles can be accessed in three different ways: (1) from the print (paper) copy; (2) from the journal's website; or (3) from an online article database like Medline. You will cite the article differently depending on how you accessed it.

Finding the journal abbreviation

Vancouver Style does not use the full journal name, only the commonly-used abbreviation: "New England Journal of Medicine" is cited as "N Engl J Med".

If the abbreviation is not stated, use the pubmed journals database to

find your journal: http://www.ncbi.nlm.nih.gov/sites/entrez?db=journals. The correct abbreviation will be listed.

Standard format for journal articles

Author Surname Initials. Title of article. Title of journal, abbreviated. Date of Publication:

Volume Number (Issue Number): Page Numbers.

Journal article in print

Haas AN, de Castro GD, Moreno T, Susin C, Albandar JM, Oppermann RV, et al. Azithromycin as a adjunctive treatment of aggressive periodontitis: 12-months randomized clinical trial. J Clin Periodontol. 2008 Aug; 35(8):696-704.

Journal article from a website

Tasdemir T, Yesilyurt C, Ceyhanli KT, Celik D, Er K. Evaluation of apical filling after root canal filling by 2 different techniques. J Can

Dent Assoc [Internet]. 2009 Apr [cited 2009 Jun 14];75(3):[about 5pp.]. Available from: http://www.cda-adc.ca/jcda/vol-75/issue-3/201.html

Journal article from an online database

Erasmus S, Luiters S, Brijlal P. Oral hygiene and dental student's knowle.g. attitude and behaviour in managing HIV/AIDS patients. Int J Dent Hyg [Internet]. 2005 Nov [cited 2009 Jun 16];3(4):213-7. Available from Medline:

http://cclsw2.vcc.ca:2048/login?url=http://search.ebscohost.com/login.aspx?direct=true&db=

cmedm&AN=16451310&site=ehost-live

Monajem S. Integration of oral health into primary health care: the role of dental hygienists and the WHO stewardship. Int J Dent Hyg [Internet]. 2006 Feb

[cited 2009 Jun 21];4(1): 47-52. Available from CINAHL with Full Text:

http://tinyurl.com/kudbxw

3. Websites

Standard format for websites

Publication information online

Publication information is often unavailable on websites and is not standardized like books or journals.

Vancouver Style requires the "Place of Publication", the "Publisher" and the "Original Publication Date" as part of the citation. If these pieces of information are not given, use: [place unknown], [publisher unknown] or [date unknown].

Author Surname Initials (if available). Title of Website [Internet]. Place of publication:

Publisher; Date of First Publication [Date of last update; cited date]. Available from: URL

Website with author

Fehrenbach MJ. Dental hygiene education [Internet]. [Place unknown]: Fehrenbach and Associates; 2000 [updated 2009 May 2; cited 2009 Jun 15]. Available from:

http://www.dhed.net/Main.html

Website without author

American Dental Hygienists' Association [Internet]. Chicago: American Dental Hygienists' Association; 2009 [cited 2009 May 30]. Available from: http://www.adha.org/

Part / Article within a website

Medline Plus [Internet]. Bethesda (MD): U.S. National Library of Medicine; c2009. Dental health; 2009 May 06 [cited 2009 Jun 16]; [about 7 screens]. Available from:

http://www.nlm.nih.gov/medlineplus/dentalhealth.html

Blog

Skariah H. The tooth booth dental blog [Internet]. Mississauga (ON): Hans Skariah; 2004-[cited 2009 Jun 20]. Available from: http://dentaldude.blogspot.com/

An Entry / article within a blog

Skariah H. The tooth booth dental blog [Internet]. Mississauga (ON): Hans Skariah; 2004 - .

Dental did you know: breastfeeding duration and non-nutritive sucking habits; 2009 May 18 [cited 2009 Jun 20]; [about 1 screen]. Available from:

http://dentaldude.blogspot.com/2009/05/dental-did-you-know-breastfeeding.html

Image on the internet

McCourtie SD, World Bank. SDM-LK-179 [image on the Internet]. 2009 Apr 29 [cited 2009 Jun 14]. Available from: http://www.flickr.com/photos/worldbank/3486672699/

Newspaper articles

Fayerman P. Women must now wait to 40 for publicly paid amnio test. Vancouver Sun. 2009 Jun 9; Sect. A:5.

Health Canada issues warning over fake toothbrushes. The Globe and Mail [Internet]. 2009 April 10 [cited 2009 Jun 23]. Available from:

http://www.theglobeandmail.com/news/national/health-canada-issues-warning-over-faketoothbrushes/ article973190/

Waldman D. Mouth is 'window on the rest of the body': oral health, dental hygiene is linked to more than teeth, gums. The National Post [Internet]. 2009 Apr 14 [cited 2009 Jun 22].

Available from Canadian Newsstand:

http://cclsw2.vcc.ca:2048/login?url=http://proquest.umi.com/pqdweb?did=1680306071&sid=1&Fmt=3&clientId=6965&RQT=309&VName=PQD

Video recordings

Dental dam: Still the best dry-field technique [DVD]. Provo (UT): Practical Clinical Courses; 2007.

Cuaron A, director; Abraham M, producer. Children of men [DVD]. Universal City (CA): Universal; 2006.

Dictionary, encyclopedia or similar reference book

Unsigned

Mosby's dental dictionary. 2nd ed. St. Louis: Mosby Elsevier; 2008. Frenotomy; p. 273.

Signed (and online)

Murchison DF. Dental emergencies. In: Merck Manual of Diagnosis and Therapy [Internet]. 18th ed. Whitehouse Station (NJ): Merck; 2009 [last modified 2009 Mar; cited 2009 Jun 23]. Available from:

http://www.merck.com/mmpe/sec08/ch096/ch096a.html?qt=dental&alt=sh

4.   Personal communications

Personal letters and conversations

Personal communications (with the exception of emails) should not be included in the Reference List, as they are unpublished and cannot be easily traced by the reader. Instead, acknowledge personal conversations and letters within the text in parentheses.

Permission

When citing any personal communication, you must have written permission from the cited person(s) to use that communication. Acknowledge the permission in a footnote or in a Notes section at the end of the text.

Conversation

"…in conversation with a fellow student from the Dental Hygiene program (Affleck, Ben. Conversation with: Matt Damon. 2008 Sep 07.).

Personal letter

"…this information was later confirmed in a letter (Hepburn, Katherine. Letter to: Spencer Tracy. 2005 Mar 03. 4 pages.).

e-mail

Email correspondence is included in the Reference List as emails are easily traceable and dated.

Bloom, Orlando. Searching Medline for dental hygiene articles [Internet]. Message to: Johnny Depp. 2008 Nov 11 [cited 2009 Jun 22]. [three paragraphs].

5. Conference paper

Unpublished paper

Surname Initial(s). Paper title. Paper presented at Name of conference; Date; Place.

Published paper

Surname author Initial(s). Paper title. In: Surname editor Initial(s), editor(s). Conference title. Place of publication: Publisher; Year. page(s).

Nørvåg K. Space-Efficient Support for Temporal Text Indexing in a Document Archive Context. In: Koch T, Sølvberg I, editors. Research and Advanced Technology for Digital Libraries. 7th European Conference, ECDL; 2003 Aug 17-22; Trondheim, Norway. Berlin: Springer; 2003. p. 511-22.

6. Newspapers and popular magazines

Surname Initial(s). Article title. Newspaper title. Date:page.

Ringen S. La ikke Erna Solberg rasere det lokale folkestyre. Aftenposten. 2004 March 25:10.

Chapter 10
MEDICAL RESEARCH WRITING

Research writing

In general, medical research writing is communicating clinical and scientific data and information to a range of audiences in a wide variety of different formats. Medical writers combine their knowledge of science and their research skills with an understanding of how to present information and pitch it at the right level for the intended audience.

Types of medical writing

- Research Protocol/ Synopsis
- Original article
- Review article
- Case report
- Case series
- Editorial
- Letter to editor
- Book review
- Dissertation
- Technical report
- Conference report
- Research grant writing

Structure of research protocol/ synopsis

The following six sections are the essential components of any medical research protocol or synopsis. These components are abbreviated

as TISTER.

T	Title
I	Introduction
S	Subjects and methods
T	Time frame and funding
E	Ethical and administrative considerations
R	References

Structure of research article

The following eight sections are the essential components of any medical article. These components are abbreviated as TAIMRDCR.

T	Title
A	Abstract
I	Introduction
M	Methods
R	Results
D	Discussion
C	Conclusion
R	References

Structure of thesis/dissertation

Dissertation

Generally for higher diplomas and not for degrees

Carries additional marks in examination

Not a criterion of success

Usually not a contribution as new knowledge

Dissertation writing

Dissertation is an **argument** to support a hypothesis

- An original piece of research
- The product of an apprenticeship
- Something that could be published

A dissertation is a must for a distinctive contribution to the knowledge of the subject and affords evidence of originality shown by the discovery of new facts and/or by the exercise of independent critical power.

- **Title**—Conveys a message
- **Abstract**—Summary of the research. May be structured or unstructured
- **Contents listing**—Shows that everything is there
- **Acknowledgements**
- **Introduction**—Statement of purpose, definitions of terms and justifications
- **Review of previous work**—Show you know the subject
- **Philosophy of the approach**—Show you can pick out an important problem
- **Plan or methodology**—Show you approached the problem in a systematic manner
- **Description of the work**—Details, so that others can follow what you did.
- **Critical analysis of the results**—Show you understand the limitations
- **Discussion and future work**—Show you know what is missing
- **Conclusions**—Most important finding in the research
- **References**—Cover the field; examiners will look for key references
- **Appendix**—The gruesome details that would clutter the description.

Title

- Concise
- Descriptive

Abstract

- A brief summary of 150–300 words
- Research question
- A rationale for the study
- The hypothesis
- The methodology
- The main findings

Introduction

- Provides a necessary background for research problems
- Begin with a general statement of the problem area
- Focus on the specific research problem
- Justification of the proposed study

Literature review

- Use subheadings to bring order
- Review of research
- Literature relevant
- Critical or just descriptive
- Comprehensive
- Link to the methodology in the thesis
- Summarize the essential aspects
- Focus, unite and cohere your discussion
- Cite influential papers
- Keep up with the recent developments

Methodology

- How do you plan to tackle the problem?
- Is there a clear hypothesis?
- Are precautions taken against bias?

- Are the limitations identified?
- Is the data collected appropriately?
- Is the methodology justified?
- Show that your approach is most appropriate.

Discussion

- Mention the limitations and weaknesses of the research.
- Compare the results with other studies.

Bibliography/ references

- Keep a database of complete references.
- Use a consistent citation style.
- Use a tool (Endnote, BibTeX, etc.).
- Attention to detail is important (correct spellings!).
- Keep complete references (page numbers, volume, location and dates for proceedings, etc.).
- Use Endnote software for reference writing.

Thesis

- Generally for degrees and not for diplomas
- Major component of exam
- Criteria of success
- Contribution as new knowledge
- Public defense

Part 1

- Title page
- Supervisor's certificate
- Dedication
- Acknowledgement
- Table of contents
- List of tables

- List of figures, graphs, illustrations
- List of abbreviations

Part 2 (about 70–100 pages)

- Abstract
- Introduction
- Review of literature
- Objective(s) of study
- Operational definitions
- Hypothesis
- Material and methods
- Result
- Discussion
- Conclusion(s)
- References (Bibliography)
- Annexes (Proforma etc.)

Most common medical writings are research article, research protocol/synopsis, and thesis/ dissertation.

WRITING A RESEARCH ARTICLE

Scientific writing is often considered a "necessary evil" to ascend the academic ladder. After all, the phrase "publish or perish" is still commonly used. Academic promotion, improving knowledge of a subject, establishing professional contacts, disseminating knowledge, and obtaining grant funding are a few reasons why physicians choose to publish.

A. Getting started

It is assumed that by now the reader has completed a well-conducted scientific study. It is time to write up the findings for a peer-reviewed scientific journal. It is always helpful to have a mentor, particularly an experienced writer in one's field who can guide. Writing an outline may seem elementary, but it can be an important tool to organize the thoughts. Deciding about the journal to publish in at

Table 10.1 Dos and don'ts for scientific manuscript writing

Section	Do	Don't
Getting started	Find a mentor. Do a thorough literature search. Make an outline. Think about journals to publish in. Think about "so what?" question for conclusion.	write down to your readers.
Abstract	Write last. Be concise.	include any data not found in the manuscript.
Introduction	Write in present tense. End with study purpose.	
Methods	Include details of what was done. Write in past tense. Include preliminary results or pilot studies. Describe the statistical analysis.	
Results	Write in past tense. Include figures and table that can be interpreted on their own. Use "signatures" to mean statistical significance.	incude citations or interpret your results Repeat data found in table in the text.
Discussion	Relate findings to your hypothesis. Interpret your statistical findings. Use past tense for your study but present tense when discussing other studies. Compare and contrast your results with other published work. Discuss the importance and clinical relevance of your findings. Discuss limitations strengths. Make suggestions for future research on your topic.	criticize other published work. come to conclusion not supported by your data. use statment such as "This is the first study to demonstrate...

the beginning is helpful as one can follow their publication guidelines as far as word count and paper structure are concerned. One should think about the conclusions of the paper before making a start to write— the "so what?" question. Why is this project novel? What makes it different from other published studies on this topic? Why is it clinically relevant? Table 1 gives a list of "dos" and "don'ts" for scientific manuscript writing.

Title

- The title of a research proposal should describe the study, be concise and inform the reader what the research is about. It reflects the objectives and design of the study. Title of the study should not contain abbreviations. It should include key words that would also help to identify appropriate reviewers. One should make it specific and captivating

'An alternative means to detect HCV'

vs

'HCV': A rapid inexpensive office screening test for early detection'

B. Writing the abstract

Although the abstract is the first writing component of a scientific manuscript, it should actually be written last. It usually requires 200-300 words. It can be structured or unstructured. A structured abstract generally has four sections: background/purpose, methods, results, and conclusions. After the rest of the paper has been completed, one can select a sentence or two from the appropriate areas (introduction, methods, results, and discussion) to include in the aforementioned abstract sections. The abstract, however, is not the introduction and should not be cut and pasted from the introduction. An abstract that is identical to the introduction in any paper or grant will be instantly rejected because of the perceived lack of effort to construct a thoughtful synthesis of the materials in the paper. One should be concise and state the purpose usually in one sentence. The emphasis should be placed on the methods and results, which should each be written in three to four sentences. The conclusion can typically be written in two sentences—the first summarizes the findings and the second makes a conclusion. Only data contained in the paper should be included in the abstract—it should not contain any new data. Care should be taken in writing the abstract. Many readers will not read past the abstract if it is not well-written. Similarly, many readers only need to scan through an abstract to determine whether an article is pertinent to their topic of interest.

C. Writing the introduction

The introduction is essentially a focused review of the pertinent existing knowledge, including published studies, project reports, and other literature. It builds an argument for conducting the study, including general and specific research objectives, the statement of the problem, and research question(s). In sum, the introduction provides a clear, succinct description of what the research is and a rationale for it. Before any writing begins, it is important to perform a thorough literature search. One should be familiar with all the recent advances in the field of study as well as important historical references. "Incomplete, inaccurate, or outdated review of the literature" is one of the common reasons for manuscript rejection. The Introduction should be written in the present tense and has the following information.

- What do you want to study? (Statement of problem)
- What has already been studied?
- What is lacking?
- What is the rationale of the study?
- What contribution will your study make?
- What are the aims/objectives?

Traditionally, the introduction is divided into four paragraphs. The first introduces the research topic and provides important definitions related to the research topic. The second paragraph gives information, incidence and prevalence of the problems or diseases. The third paragraph describes the rationale of the research. The last paragraph is about goals, aims and objectives of the study and should end with the purpose: a hypothesis of what one is expecting to find. In short, the introduction describes what is already known, what is unknown and why one wants to know.

D. Writing the materials and methods

The traditional sequence of a manuscript is introduction, methods, results, and discussion, which has been referred to by the acronym IMRAD. Pollock et al. have suggested drafting the manuscript in the sequence MRDAI. Author's preferred sequence is writing methods first, followed by results. Discussion and introduction sections are written at the same time. The methods section should be written in enough detail that another researcher would be able to duplicate the study. In fact, the methods section is most often responsible for outright rejection of a manuscript because the lack of detail is a common problem. This is the section where one should state everything one did (controlling for biases, validating research tools) to increase the reliability of the results.

The Methods section should be written in the past tense. If it is a study involving human subjects, one should obtain the institutional review board's approval and state it. Subject inclusion and exclusion criteria should be mentioned. One should also take account of how and from where subjects were recruited, as well as randomization and blinding procedures. Including patient characteristics, such as disease stage or severity and comorbid conditions can help the readers to determine whether the findings of the article are applicable to their patients of interest.

It may be helpful to include a diagram of the number of subjects recruited, how many were excluded, losses to follow- up or withdrawal, and your final sample size. Details of the sample are included in the results, but most journals will require that the previously stated

information is included in the methods. Likewise, preliminary experiments or pilot studies can be included in the methods section if they helped to arrive at the methods used in the study.

If equipment was used, the equipment manufacturer, model, and calibration methods should be included. It may also be helpful to include a timeline that shows how and when different aspects of the study protocol took place. The final paragraph of the methods section should describe the statistical analysis. The tests used, the p value that determined statistical significance, and whether an a priori power analysis was conducted to decide the necessary sample size should be mentioned.

The power and sample size calculation is often a neglected area of scientific presentation and should always be performed before conducting a study.

E. Writing the results

In writing the results section, it is important to "only state the facts!" The Results section is not a place to include citations or the interpretation of the data. One should make one's point with data, not arguments. The results section should be written in the past tense.

One should begin by describing the study sample demographic data, which can be done in a simple table. The data reported in a table should not be repeated in the text. Furthermore, tables and figures should stand on their own. One should include a title, legend, and labels for the axes. The readers should be able to determine what the table is about by only looking at it and not having to read any text. Any percentages should include raw numbers so that the readers are not misled by a large percentage (such as 25 percent) that only came from one of four subjects.

It should be noted that the word "significance" should only be used to describe statistical significance. One should avoid using significant as a synonym for importance. General phrases, such as "showed a trend toward" when results are not statistically significant, often tend to signal a poor study design and should be avoided. Also, the word "data" is plural. Thus, it is correct to state, "Our data are . . ." rather than "Our data is...."

F. Writing the discussion

One should begin writing the discussion by discussing the major findings and relating them to the hypothesis. Was the null hypothesis rejected or was it expected? Although being unable to reject the null hypothesis (for example, seeing no significant change between the treatment groups) may seem like a "crash and burn" situation, one can still publish the paper.

Generally manuscripts describing studies with negative findings are especially tough to get accepted by medical journals, with publication rates generally less than one-third that of manuscripts describing studies with positive findings.

One should mention priori power analysis to determine the necessary sample size to avoid a beta error (concluding that there is no difference between treatment groups when there is in fact a difference). Previous studies have shown that physicians, particularly those with no formal education in epidemiology and biostatistics, have a limited ability to interpret study results.

More than 58 percent of medical residents, however, use statistical information in the published literature in forming opinions or when making medical decisions. Thus, it is important in the discussion to spell out the meaning of the statistical findings without appearing arrogant to your readers.

When describing the study, past tense should be used, but present tense should be used for established knowledge from other investigators. One should compare and contrast the results to those found in the literature. Care should be taken not to criticize other published work. Similar findings will strengthen the results, but one should still point out how the study differs from previous similar studies.

When explaining the study results, it is important to consider all possible explanations rather than just those that fit the preconceived biases. One should, however, avoid coming to conclusions that are not supported by the data. Some of the most common criticisms of the Discussion section by editors and reviewers involve coming to erroneous or unsupported conclusions, drawing conclusions disproportionate to the results, uncritically accepting statistical results, and interpreting the findings in a manner not concordant with data reported.

Unless one is absolutely sure that it is true, one should avoid statements such as, "This is the first study to demonstrate... .." After all, there are few studies that change the course of scientific progress, but some authors are overly enthusiastic in advertising their study as a seminal contribution. It is also important to discuss the clinical relevance of the findings and how patients or physicians may benefit from them. Describing confidence intervals is really helpful in this regard.

In the discussion section, it is essential to address the limitations and strengths of the study. I have stated them in this order, rather than as strengths and limitations, because it is nice to leave the reader on a good note when he or she finishes reading the paper. Thus, acknowledge the study's limitations first.

One limitation may include a lack of generalizability, which often happens when trying to obtain a homogeneous sample. One may use the study's limitations to make suggestions for future research. If not, one should still include suggestions for further research, usually in the concluding section.

This last paragraph or last few sentences can also be used to propose ideas for changes to medical practice.

G. Remembering style and grace

Throughout the writing and editing process, it is important to remember the style and grace that is needed in writing any good manuscript.

First of all, do not make the readers and reviewers work unnecessarily! When reading through the paper, try to keep the reviewers in mind. When a question is left unanswered or is not answered until the discussion, the readers can get frustrated and give up on the paper entirely. Consistently use the same word to describe the same thing to provide continuity and avoid confusion.

Of course, it is also helpful to have someone else read your manuscript—a colleague and maybe even a layperson. A different set of eyes and a different perspective can point out areas that need clarity. Use transitions for flow. Transitions let the reader know how each sentence relates to the story and how parts of sentences are related. One should also limit the use of passive language. Although scientists tend to use it because they think that it is objective and do not want to indicate who is conducting a certain action, it becomes quite boring to continually read, "The sutures were removed" and "The data were analyzed."

One should avoid wordiness and using long or unfamiliar words when a commonly used shorter one will convey the same message. Words such as marked, revealed, and demonstrated are overused and have lost their intended meaning. Although it is common for writers, especially inexperienced ones, to try to use "flowery" language, it is best to remember that "less is more." One can delete unnecessary adjectives and adverbs, such as 'fundamentally', 'very', and 'great'. The words 'while' and 'since' have primary temporal definitions, but 'while' is often used as a synonym for 'although' or 'whereas' and 'since' is commonly used instead of 'because'"

Be mindful of the fine points that can slow down the readers and cause them to misinterpret what one is trying to say. Well-written paragraphs usually start with making a point in the first sentence and then developing that point throughout the paragraph. Focusing on a single major point in each paragraph allows the readers to follow the author's train of thought.

H. General reminders

There are a few other general reminders to keep in mind. Follow the journal guidelines as far as formatting, line numbering, word limits, figures, and citations. This will save the time and hassle of having the editor send the paper back before it can be sent out for review. If there are large blocks of text, it might be a good idea to add one or more subheadings.

Make sure that the font is the same throughout and that italics are not overused. Some reviewers do not like to see italics because the overuse of italics may signal to the reviewers that the authors consider the materials presented to be too complex for the reviewers to understand.

Spell out abbreviations the first time one uses them but do not try to avoid word count limitations by bombarding the readers with multiple abbreviations. Non-universal abbreviations force the readers to remember their meanings and substitute the full phrase each time they appear. An abbreviation should be used often enough in the paper, preferably more than 10 times, so that the readers do not forget the meaning.

Of course, proofread, proofread, proofread, and use spell check! As previously mentioned, allow someone else to proofread, too. One should also look through one's final manuscript and notice the citations. Make sure that one is citing a wide range of authors and not repeating someone else's ideas. Although one should be optimistic, one should also remember that there is a chance that the manuscript will be rejected by the journal.

The acceptance rate of clinical research-based manuscripts submitted to major biomedical journals is 30 to 40 percent. The acceptance rate for journals such as the *New England Journal of Medicine* and *JAMA* is less than 10 percent. Even if the manuscript is not accepted, the comments by the reviewers will most likely help to identify the weaknesses and improve the paper. If manuscript is accepted with revisions (major or minor), then congratulations!

In revising, one should draft a response letter with each reviewer's comments typed out and explain how they have been addressed. Also state where in the paper the revision can be found (i.e. methods section, paragraph 2, line 2). Remember to be polite; if one is choosing not to make a suggested revision, a reason for not doing so should be given. Although it is not necessary to do every suggested change, but remember the manuscript will not be looked upon kindly if one chooses to make a rebuttal for all or the majority of suggestions.

Although scientific writing can be a long and tedious process, the writing ability will continuously improve. Remember, only the researcher who is competent in the art of written communication can play an active and effective role in contributing to science.

Research protocol/synopsis writing

Writing a title and introduction is the same as of a research article. However, in the introduction the researcher has to sell his idea and more emphasis is put on 'so what' component of the introduction. It becomes a 'sales document' designed to convince the readers that the proposed work should be considered for endorsement and support.

It provides you an opportunity to convince the reviewers that you are up-to-date and conversant in your field of enquiry. You should provide a concise, thorough, well referenced review. Preliminary data may strengthen your proposal. The last paragraph should lead to the logical conclusion that your proposed question needs to be answered.

Introduction is followed by the heading **Objective/s** and after writing the objective in future tense the researcher gives the appropriate **operational definitions** if required.

Hypothesis is stated after the operational definitions.

The methodology of a research proposal documents how and when the research will be conducted. It is the most detailed part of the proposal. It is written in the future tense. The major difference from a research article is that separate headings are given and include:

- Study design
- Study setting
- Duration of study
- Study population
- Study instruments
- Sampling: (design, frame, size). The number of subjects/objects should be the key to the minimum necessary for valid results
- Criteria of selection of subjects (inclusion and exclusion criteria)
- Data collection procedure
- Analysis and presentation plan including appropriate statistics according to the variables under study should be mentioned
- Ethical considerations

The other major difference is that **scheduling/phasing** of the proposed research should be given in the form of Gantt charts.

Chapter

11

RESEARCH ETHICS

The first step in the evolution of ethics is a sense of solidarity with other human beings. (Albert Schweitzer)

Definition

Research ethics are defined as guidelines for the responsible conduct of biomedical research including safety of the researcher, subjects and contribute to the good of society. In addition, research ethics educates and monitors scientists conducting research to ensure a high ethical standard.

Brief history

The birth of modern research ethics began with a desire to protect human subjects involved in research projects. The first attempt to craft regulations began during the Doctors Trial of 1946-1947. The Doctors Trial was a segment of the Nuremberg Trials for Nazi war criminals. In the Doctors Trial, 23 German Nazi physicians were accused of conducting torturous experiments with concentration camp inmates. The accused physicians tortured, brutalized, crippled, and murdered thousands of victims in the name of research. Some of their experiments involved gathering scientific information about the limits of the human body by exposing victims to extreme temperatures and altitudes. The most gruesome and destructive experiments tested how quickly a human could be euthanatized in

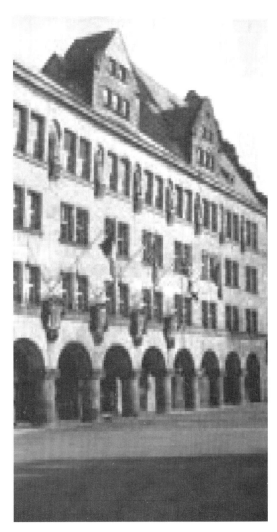

Fig.11.1 Nuremberg palace

(Photo of the Nuremberg Palace of Justice; Photo by Thomas J. Dodd Papers, Dodd Research Center, University Libraries, University of Connecticut)

order to carry out the Nazi racial purification policies most efficiently.

To prosecute the accused Nazi doctors for the atrocities they committed, a list of ethical guidelines for the conduct of research—the **Nuremberg code** was constituted.

The Nuremberg Code consisted of ten basic ethical principles that the accused violated.

The 10 guidelines were as follows:

1. Research participants must voluntarily consent to research participation.
2. Research aims should contribute to the good of society.
3. Research must be based on sound theory and prior animal testing.
4. Research must avoid unnecessary physical and mental suffering.
5. No research projects can go forward where serious injury and/or death are potential outcomes.
6. The degree of risk taken with research participants cannot exceed anticipated benefits of results.
7. Proper environment and protection for participants is necessary.
8. Experiments can be conducted only by scientifically qualified persons.
9. Human subjects must be allowed to discontinue their participation at any time.
10. Scientists must be prepared to terminate the experiment if there is cause to believe that continuation will be harmful or result in injury or death.

The Nuremberg Guidelines paved the way for the next major initiative designed to promote responsible research with human subjects, the **Helsinki declaration**. The Helsinki Declaration was developed by the World Medical Association and has been revised and updated periodically since 1964. The document lays out basic ethical principles for conducting biomedical research and specifies guidelines for research conducted either by a physician, in conjunction with medical care, or within a clinical setting.

The Helsinki Declaration contains all the basic ethical elements specified in the Nuremberg Code but then advances further guidelines specifically designed to address the unique vulnerabilities of human subjects solicited to participate in clinical research projects. The unique principles developed within the Declaration include:

• The necessity of using an independent investigator to review potential research projects.

• Employing a medically qualified person to supervise the research and assume responsibility for the health and welfare of human subjects.

• The importance of preserving the accuracy of research results.

• Suggestions on how to obtain informed consent from research participants.

• Rules concerning research with children and mentally incompetent persons.

• Evaluating and using experimental treatments on patients.

• The importance of determining which medical situations and conditions are appropriate and safe for research.

Following the Helsinki Declaration, the next set of research ethics guidelines came out in the **Belmont report** of 1979, from the National Commission for the Protection of Human Subjects of Biomedical and Behavioral Research. The report outlines:

1. The ethical principles for research with human subjects.
2. Boundaries between medical practice and research.
3. The concepts of respect for persons, beneficence, and justice.
4. Applications of these principles in informed consent (respect for persons),

assessing risks and benefits (beneficence), and subject selection (justice).

The Nuremberg, Helsinki, and Belmont guidelines provided the foundation of more ethically uniform research to which stringent rules and consequences for violation were attached. Governmental laws and regulations concerning the responsible conduct of research have since been developed for research that involves both human and animal subjects. The **Animal Welfare Act** provides guidelines and regulations for research with animals. It goes into detail about sale, licensure, facilities, transport, and other care instructions.

IRB

For research with human subjects, **Title 45, part 46 from the code of federal regulations (45 CFR 46): The protection of human subjects regulations** outlines the purpose and policies of **Institutional review board (IRB)** oversight and approval, informed consent, and protections and policies for research with children, pregnant women, fetuses, prisoners, and mentally incompetent individuals.

Currently, the focus of research ethics lies in the education of researchers regarding the ethical principles behind regulations as well as the oversight and review of current and potential research projects. The field has expanded from providing protections for human subjects to including ethical guidelines that encompass all parts of research from research design to the truthful reporting of results.

There are several avenues for people who wish to seek education on basic ethical principles, and avenues for education on how to comply with policies at the institutional, state, and national levels. The University of Minnesota's Center for Bioethics (www.bioethics.umn.edu) and many other universities and professional associations around the country continually offer education for researchers and scientists on ethical research issues.

Values in medical ethics

Six of the values that commonly apply to medical ethics discussions are:

5. **Autonomy**—The patient has the right to refuse or choose their treatment.
6. **Beneficence**—A practitioner should act in the best interest of the patient.
7. **Nonmaleficence**—First, "do no harm".
8. **Justice**—Concerns the distribution of scarce health resources, and the decision of who gets what treatment.
9. **Dignity**—The patient (and the person treating the patient) have the right to dignity.
10. **Truthfulness and honesty**—The concept of informed consent has increased in importance since the historical events of the doctors' trial of the Nuremberg trials and the Tuskegee syphilis study.

Why study research ethics?

Knowing what constitutes ethical research is important for all people who conduct research projects or use and apply the results from research findings. All researchers should be familiar with the basic ethical principles and have up-to-date knowledge about policies and procedures designed to ensure the safety of research subjects and to prevent sloppy or irresponsible research, because ignorance of policies designed to protect research subjects is not considered a viable excuse for ethically questionable projects. Therefore, the duty lies with the researcher to seek out and fully understand the policies and theories designed to guarantee upstanding research practices. The examples of unethical research are as follows:

- **Tuskegee experiment** (1932-1972):

American researchers purposely withheld treatment for 399 African-American people with syphilis for the sole purpose of studying the long term effects of the disease.

- **Willowbrook study** (1963-1966): Children with developmental disabilities were deliberately infected with Hepatitis (some were even fed fecal matter). Purpose of the study was to examine the course of the disease and to test a potential immunization.

- Human radiation experiments by the **US Department of defense and atomic energy commission**

- **Milgram's obedience study:** Researchers asked participants to "Pseudo-shocking" confederates in order to examine obedience.

- **Zimbardo-Stanford prison experiment** (1971): Study had to end prematurely because of abusive behaviors generated in participants who where assigned as guards over those subjects who were assigned as prisoners.

Research is a public trust that must be ethically conducted, trustworthy, and socially responsible if the results are to be valuable. All parts of a research project – from the project design to submission of the results for peer review – have to be upstanding in order to be considered ethical. When even one part of a research project is questionable or conducted unethically, the integrity of the entire project is called into question.

1. Save the vulnerable populations

There is always an ethical concern when recruiting from vulnerable populations:

- Poor; homeless
- Mentally ill
- Terminally ill
- Prisoners
- Students
- Staff

Avoid an exploitative transaction

An exploitative transaction is one in which person 'A' takes unfair advantage of person 'B' (Wertheimer, 1999).

Research fraud and authorship

is the process of deciding whose names belong on a research paper. In many cases, research evolves from collaboration and assistance between experts and colleagues. Some of this assistance will require acknowledgement and some will require joint authorship.

Responsible authorship practices are an important part of research. Reporting and analyzing results is the key to applying research findings to the real world. Despite its vital role, authorship remains a murky and vague area for many scientists who frequently run into difficulty when deciding which colleagues should be listed as authors or coauthors, and which colleagues should instead receive acknowledgement. Despite the challenges, researchers should familiarize themselves with proper authorship practices in order to protect their work and ideas while also preventing research fraud.

Ethical guidelines for authorship

Each person listed as an author on an article should have significantly contributed to both the research and writing. In addition, all listed authors must be prepared to accept full responsibility for the content of the research article. The International Committee of Medical Journal Editors (ICMJE) is the recognized international expert organization when it comes to guidelines regarding biomedical research authorship. Their website (www.icmje.org) lists all requirements for authorship, which are quoted as follows:

Authorship credit should be based only on

1. substantial contributions to conception and design, or acquisition of data, or analysis and interpretation of data;

2. drafting the article or revising it critically for important intellectual content;

3. final approval of the version.

Who can be a co-author?

A co-author is someone who has

1. contributed substantially to the research, AND

2. wrote or revised all or part of the manuscript, AND

3. Approved the final version of the entire article.

According to the ICMJE, colleagues who are part of a research group or team but do not meet the conditions above should not be listed as authors. They should instead receive acknowledgement at the end of the manuscript, with a brief description of their contribution if appropriate. In order to acknowledge a contributing colleague, the colleague must consent to the acknowledgement, lest they seem to be endorsing research or conclusions drawn from research for which they are not responsible.

All the contributing co-authors of an article must jointly decide the order of the listing of names. The first person listed should be the person most closely involved with the research. The authors should then decide the order of the remaining authors in accordance with the criteria of the publishing journal.

Plagiarism is the act of passing off somebody else's ideas, thoughts, pictures, theories, words, or stories as your own. If a researcher plagiarizes the work of others, they are bringing into question the integrity, ethics, and trustworthiness of the sum total of his or her research. In addition, plagiarism is both an illegal act and punishable, considered to be on the same level as stealing from the author that which he or she originally created.

Plagiarism takes many forms. On one end of the spectrum are people who intentionally take a passage word-for-word, put it in their own work, and do not properly credit the original author. The other end consists of unintentional (or simply lazy) paraphrased and fragmented texts the author has pieced together from several works without properly citing the original sources. No parts of the spectrum of potential plagiaristic acts are tolerated by the scientific community, and research manuscripts will be rejected by publishers if they contain any form of plagiarism–including unintentional plagiarism.

Ethical guidelines to avoid plagiarism

The Indiana University website provides the following advice to avoid plagiarism.

A researcher preparing a written manuscript should cite the original source if he or she:

* Quotes another person's actual words, either oral or written;

* Paraphrases another person's words, either oral or written;

* Uses another person's idea, opinion, or theory; or

* Borrows facts, statistics, or other illustrative material, unless the information is common knowledge.

The rules of plagiarism typically apply to graphics, text, and other visuals from all traditional forms of publication and include modern forms of publication as well, in particular the world wide web. If a substantial amount of another person's graphics or text will be lifted from a web page, an author should ask permission to use the material from the original author or website host.

Most researchers certainly try not to plagiarize. However, it isn't always easy because people often consult a variety of sources of information for their research and end up mixing it in with their own background knowledge. To avoid unintentional or accidental plagiarizing of another person's work, use the following tips from the Northwestern University website:

• Cite all ideas and information that is not your own and/or is not common knowledge.

• Always use quotation marks if you are using someone else's words.

• At the beginning of a paraphrased section, show that what comes next is someone else's original idea (example: these bullet points start out by saying the information originated with Northwestern University).

• At the end of a paraphrased section, place the proper citation.

Redundant publications constitute a special type of plagiarism. The ICMJE defines redundant publication as follows:

"Redundant or duplicate publication is publication of a paper that overlaps substantially with one already published."

Peer review is the process in which an author (or authors) submits a written manuscript or article to a journal for publication and the journal editor distributes the article to experts working in the same, or similar, scientific discipline. The experts, otherwise called the reviewers, and the editor then enter the peer review process. The process involves the following:

1. Reviewers and editors read and evaluate the article.

2. Reviewers submit their reviews back to the journal editor.

3. The journal editor takes all comments, including their own, and communicates this feedback to the original author (or authors).

The peer review process seldom proceeds in a straight line. The entire process may involve several rounds of communication between the editor, the reviewers, and the original author (or authors) before an article is fully ready for publication.

According to an article on quality peer reviews in the *Journal of the American Medical Association*, a high quality peer review should evaluate a biomedical article or publication on the following merits:

• Importance—Does the research impact health and health care?

• Usefulness—Does the study provide useful scientific information?

• Relevance—Does the research apply to the journal's readers and content area of interest?

• Sound methods—Was the research conducted with sound scientific methods that allowed the researchers to answer their research question?

• Sound ethics—Was the study conducted ethically ensuring proper protection for human subjects? Were results reported accurately and honestly?

• Completeness—Is all information relevant to the study included in the article?

• Accuracy—Is the written product a true reflection of the conduct and results of the research?

Ethical guidelines for peer review

The two most important ethical concepts in the peer review process are confidentiality and protection of intellectual property. Reviewers should not know the author (or authors) they are reviewing, and the author (or authors) should not be told the names of the reviewers. Only by maintaining strict confidentiality guidelines can the peer review process be truly open and beneficial. Likewise, no person involved in the peer review process – either the editor, reviewers, or other journal staff – can publicly disclose the information in the article or use the information in a submitted article for personal gain.

Peer reviewers, in addition to maintaining confidentiality, can be neither conflicted nor political in their review. Conflicts may take the form of financial conflicts with the results, conflicts if the research is too similar to their own research endeavors, and conflicts due to personal relationships with the author (or authors). Political motivations that might interfere with the peer review process include competition to publish with other scientists and inaccurate reviews designed to "punish" a competing colleague or journal.

Editors may find it difficult to guarantee a conflict-free peer review process, because reviewers must be experts with knowledge unique to the field to which the article pertains. Therefore, many reviewers may find themselves faced with an article concerning research that is very similar to their own. Peer reviewers should disclose all conflicts of interest that may unduly influence their review to the journal editor and disqualify themselves when appropriate.

Editors of journals should maintain an open and ethical peer review process, and all submitting authors and readers should be fully aware of a journal's process of peer review. Editors do retain flexibility in assigning the number of peer reviewers and what to do with the peer review information once completed. One method is for an editor to approach two or three reviewers and then ask an author (or authors) to change the article to satisfy all the reviews. On the other hand, an editor may take all the reviews and consolidate the advice to help guide the author (or authors) when making changes, clarifications, and corrections. Editors must not relinquish too many of their own responsibilities to peer reviewers. The peer review process represents one step in the publishing process and editors

need to take full responsibility for their decision to include an article in their journal. This means that editors must review the content and character of a submitted article, using all the criteria listed for reviewers above, and should rely on the reviewers primarily to catch errors that lie outside the editor's area of expertise and technical understanding.

Finally, editors should have full and complete freedom over the content of a published journal. They should only include articles that they believe to be honest, accurate, ethical, and scientifically responsible.

Conflicts of interest arise when a person's (or an organization's) obligations to a particular research project conflict with their personal interests or obligations. For example, a university researcher who owns stock in XYZ Pharmaceuticals is obligated to report truthful and accurate data, but he might be conflicted if faced with data that would hurt stock prices for XYZ pharmaceuticals. Conflicts of interest are particularly important to examine within the context of biomedical research because research subjects may be particularly vulnerable to harm.

A researcher should attempt to identify potential conflicts of interest in order to confront those issues before they have a chance to do harm or damage. If conflicts of interest do exist, then the objectivity of the researcher and the integrity of the research results can be questioned by any person throughout the research review process – from the IRB review through the peer review phase. It is therefore imperative to address conflicts of interest up front and discuss how to combat potential lack of objectivity, before the research is called into question.

Ethical guidelines for conflicts of interest

The "Objectivity in Research NIH Guide," provides guidelines on how investigators receiving grants from the National Institutes of Health (NIH) should handle conflicts of interest. In essence, it suggests that investigators and organizations should:

- Disclose to their institution any major or significant financial conflicts of interest that might interfere with their ability to conduct a research project objectively.

- Disclose any such financial conflicts of interest of their spouses or dependent Children.

- The organization must have, a written and enforced administrative process to identify and manage, reduce, or eliminate conflicting financial interests with respect to research projects for which NIH funding is sought.

- Before any NIH funds are spent, the organization must inform the Chief Grants Management Officer (CGMO) at the appropriate NIH office of any existing conflicts of interest and indicate that the conflict has been addressed, "by indicating whether the conflict has either been managed, reduced, or eliminated;"

- The organization has to identify and report any conflicts that arise during the course of NIH funded research;

- The organization has to comply with NIH requests for information on how an identified conflict of interest has been handled.

- The NIH recommends the following possible actions to help organizations address conflicts of interest:

- Public disclosure of significant financial interests;

- Monitoring of research by independent reviewers;

- Modification of the research plan;

- Disqualification from participation in all or a portion of the research funded by PHS;

- Divestiture of significant financial interests; or

- Severance of relationships that create actual or potential conflicts."

Physicians and other healthcare professional researchers may find themselves facing conflicts of interest in their duties towards research versus their duties towards the health and welfare of their patients. Clinical obligations to patients should always be considered above and beyond the obligations of research.

Ethical guidelines for data management: In respect to research ethics, there are three issues:

1. The ethical and truthful collection of reliable data

2. The ownership and responsibility of collected data

3. Retaining data and sharing access to collected data with colleagues and the public

Each issue contributes to the integrity of research and can be easily overlooked by researchers. It is not adequate research practice to assume issues involved in data collection will work themselves out on their own. Instead, a clear, responsible, ethically sound, and carefully outlined plan for data management is required at the beginning of research to prevent all manners of conflicts and inappropriate research methods.

Ethical data collection refers to collecting data in a way that does not harm or injure someone. Harm and injury could range from outright physical injury to harmful disclosure of unprotected confidential health information. In comparison, truthful data collection refers to data that, once collected, are not manipulated or altered in any way that might impact or falsely influence results.

Assigning and ensuring responsibility for collecting and maintaining data is one of the most important ethical considerations when conducting a research project.

Responsibilities include the following important issues:

- Oversight of the design of the method of data collection.
- Protecting research subjects from harm.
- Securing and storing data safely to preserve the integrity and privacy of data.
- Delegating work with data to others and responsibility over the work of others.
- Responsible use of data and truthful portrayal of data results.

In contrast to the fairly straightforward concepts underlying truthful and ethical data collection issues, the issue of data sharing is complicated by personal emotions, motives, obligations, and ownership. Despite its complexities, data sharing is considered to be a hallmark of the scientific community, particularly in academia. NIH describes the importance of data sharing on its website:

Data sharing achieves many important goals for the scientific community, such as reinforcing open scientific inquiry, encouraging diversity of analysis and opinion, promoting new research, testing of new or alternative hypothesis and methods of analysis, supporting studies on data collection methods and measurement, facilitating teaching of new researchers, enabling the exploration of topics not envisioned by the initial investigators, and permitting the creation of new data sets by combining data from multiple sources.

While part of scientific research encourages accuracy and verification of data through data sharing, sometimes data are associated with intellectual property and need to be protected as such. For this reason, whether to retain or share data can be a fine line for researchers who wish to protect their intellectual property, but the line must be properly drawn in order to allow the positive aspects of data sharing to occur while protecting the researcher's hard work and ingenuity.

The three issues for data management (ethical and truthful data collection, responsibility of collected data, and data sharing) can be addressed by researchers before and during the establishment of a new research project. Researchers must accurately identify answers to the following questions to resolve and address all data management issues in a timely manner:

- Who is in charge of the data? (This person is usually the principal investigator of the research project and is responsible for data collection design and physical data collection).
- How will data be collected? (Will data be collected via phone, mail, personal interview, existing records, secondary sources, etc.)?
- Will there be identifying information within the data? If yes, why? How will this be rectified?
- How will data be stored and what privacy and protection issues will result from the method of storage? (Will it be stored electronically, on paper, as raw tissue samples, etc.)?
- Who will ensure that no data were excluded from the final results and ensure accuracy of result interpretation?
- How long after the project is over will data be kept? (This will depend on the source of funding and organizational policies).

Protecting intellectual property while at the same time encouraging data sharing is highly important in order to ensure valid and reliable research. In order to identify what is and is not protected as "intellectual property," the concept must be clearly defined. The University of Minnesota's Intellectual Property Policy defines intellectual property as:

'Intellectual Property' means any invention,

discovery, improvement, copyrightable work, integrated circuit mask work, trademark, trade secret, and licensable know-how and related rights. Intellectual property includes, but is not limited to, individual or multimedia works of art or music, records of confidential information generated or maintained by the University, data, texts, instructional materials, tests, bibliographies, research findings, organisms, cells, viruses, DNA sequences, other biological materials, probes, crystallographic coordinates, plant lines, chemical compounds, and theses.★ Intellectual property may exist in a written or electronic form, may be raw or derived, and may be in the form of text, multimedia, computer programs, spreadsheets, formatted fields in records or forms within files, databases, graphics, digital images, video and audio recordings, live video or audio broadcasts, performances, two or three-dimensional works of art, musical compositions, executions of processes, film, film strips, slides, charts, transparencies, other visual/aural aids or CD-ROMS.

NIH guidelines on data sharing. The primary guideline states that all data must be shared and released in a timely manner. The NIH defines timely manner as no later than acceptance for publication. In addition, all grant applications to the NIH for grants of at least $500,000 are required to establish a data sharing plan or give an explanation as to why data will not be shared in the proposal (i.e. IRB allowance or institutional restrictions).

The Health Information Portability and Accountability Act (HIPAA) It provides detailed guidelines about data sharing and using data containing personal identification information. The HIPAA guidelines protect personal health information and provide legal requirements for all segments of the health care system (including biomedical research) concerning what type of information can be shared, how information should be stored and protected, data coding, and how information

is used. Genetic information is an area of particular concern when considering the issues surrounding data management. Due to the wealth of information locked inside the human genome and the potential for using this information to determine a variety of conditions and genetic tendencies, including the potential to identify a person based on his or her genetic information, particular interest has been expressed in protecting the information found in DNA. Careful attention should be paid by researchers when using genetic information due to its sensitive nature.

Research misconduct is the process of identifying and reporting unethical or unsound research. Research misconduct is defined as fabrication, falsification, or plagiarism in proposing, performing, or reviewing research, or in reporting research results.

- **Fabrication** is making up data or results and recording or reporting them.

- **Falsification** is manipulating research materials, equipment, or processes, or changing or omitting data or results such that the research is not accurately represented in the research record.

- **Plagiarism** is the appropriation of another person's ideas, processes, results, or words without giving appropriate credit.

- **Research misconduct** does not include honest error or differences of opinion.

In addition to defining research misconduct includes guidelines on what must be present in order to find a researcher guilty of committing research misconduct.

A finding of research misconduct requires that:

- There be a significant departure from accepted practices of the relevant research community; and

- The misconduct be committed intentionally, or knowingly, or recklessly; and

- The allegation be proven by a preponderance of evidence.

Research misconduct can be the result of criminal behavior. For example, making up research data that doesn't exist and other overt acts of fraud are deliberate and punishable criminal acts. Government regulations and criminal punishments are necessary to prevent these criminal practices. Research misconduct can also be the result of mistaken, negligent, unintentional, lazy, or sloppy research practices. These types of misconduct are usually covered by institutional policies and are punishable at the institutional level. In these instances of research misconduct, the use of outside research evaluators (like the IRB) and the process of peer review help to maintain and safeguard scientific integrity.

Ethical guidelines for research misconduct

Who is responsible for reviewing instances of research misconduct? Any person who knows that research is being conducted unethically should raise his or her concerns to the appropriate authorities, whether that person is involved in the research or not. The first step in this instance may likely be a confidential conversation with the person in charge of research integrity at an institution. Once research misconduct has been identified, all parties involved in the research must take responsibility to resolve the situation, including: the principal investigator, co-investigators, the institution hosting the research, the funding agency, and publishing journal editors, if applicable. While the federal government takes responsibility for research projects funded with federal money, it assigns the primary responsibilities of identifying and investigating research misconduct to the agency or institution hosting the research.

Research with animals

Animals play a significant role in research. They are used in a variety of ways by researchers, such as for testing new pharmaceuticals, as teaching tools for medical students, and as experimental subjects for new surgical procedures. Research with animals is necessary and vital to biomedical research because animal research is frequently a necessary first step towards research involving new medical treatments and pharmaceuticals intended for human use.

Many dedicated organizations and individuals are interested in protecting and safeguarding animal subjects as regards their use in research. Some organizations are interested in eliminating the use of animals in research. Others consider research with animals a necessary evil to the advancement of medicine, but still aim to eliminate unnecessary suffering, pain, and poor facility conditions for animal subjects.

To protect animals, research projects that use animals have to be reviewed. These review processes assess the risks and benefits of using animals in research. This can prove difficult for project reviewers and often makes for intense debates and arguments about the appropriate use of animal subjects, particularly because the animal subjects usually bear all the risks while human beings realize all the benefits. Debates also center on judging how much pain is too much, whether or not animals experience pain in the same way that humans do, and whether or not these ideas should even factor into the debate at all.

To assure that research with animals is conducted ethically and responsibly, the federal government has created regulations involving the use and care of animals involved in teaching, testing, and research.

Ethical guidelines for animal research

In order to prevent the mistreatment of animals the United States government first passed the Animal Welfare Act in 1966. The Animal Welfare Act exists in order:

1. To insure that animals intended for use in research facilities or for exhibition purposes or for use as pets are provided humane care and treatment;

2. to assure the humane treatment of animals during transportation in commerce;

3. to protect the owners of animals from the theft of their animals by preventing the sale or use of animals which have been stolen.

The responsibility for enforcing the Animal Welfare Act and protecting animals used in testing, teaching, and research falls on a number of different shoulders.

Research with human subjects

The issues concerning research with human subjects involves topics ranging from voluntary participation in research to fair selection and justice. This variety makes the topics surrounding research ethics with human subjects a challenging but important charge.

Respect for persons—Informed consent. Informed consent exists to ensure that all research involving human subjects allows for voluntary participation by subjects who understand what participation entails. **Informed consent** means that people approached and asked to participate in a research study must: a) know what they are getting involved with before they commit; b) not be coerced or manipulated in any way to participate; and, c) must consent to participate in the project as a subject.

The Belmont report of 1979, outlines the three requirements for informed consent. The first requirement is that information disclosed to research participants must include, "research procedure, their purposes, risks and anticipated benefits, alternative procedures (where therapy is involved), and a statement offering the subject the opportunity to ask questions and to withdraw at any time from the research."

The second requirement for informed consent is comprehension. The concept of comprehension requires researchers to adapt information to be understandable to every participant. This requires taking into consideration different abilities, intelligence levels, maturity, and language needs.

Finally, the third requirement for informed consent is **voluntariness**. Informed consent can be neither coerced nor improperly pressured from any participant.

Respect for persons–Privacy and confidentiality. Privacy and confidentiality are very important components for research involving human subjects. People have a right to protect themselves, and information gathered during research participation could harm a person by violating their right to keep information about themselves private. The information gathered from people in biomedical studies has a unique potential to be particularly embarrassing, harmful, or damaging.

Recently, a number of research projects have focused on unlocking genetic information. Genetic information may violate a person's right to privacy if not adequately protected. The very fact that genetic information contains information about identity provides a unique challenge to researchers. Many genetic experiments may seem harmless, but during the process of collecting genetic information on, for example, breast cancer, a researcher will inevitably collect a wealth of other identifiable information that could potentially be linked to research participants as well.

The health information portability and accountability act (HIPAA)

There are two main provisions in HIPAA. The first provision prevents workers and their families from losing health insurance when changing jobs.

The second part of HIPAA is the Administrative Simplification Compliance Act (ASCA) and this part identifies issues in health information privacy and confidentiality. ASCA contains strict regulations concerning health information privacy, security (particularly of electronically stored health data), and personal identifiers attached to data. This is the strictest step taken thus far by the federal government to protect the vast amount of personal electronic health information maintained by health insurance companies, hospitals, clinics, researchers, and the government. It is governed by the following principles:

Risk benefit and beneficence. Beneficence is a principle used frequently in research ethics. It means, "doing good." Biomedical research strives to do good by studying diseases and health data to uncover information that may be used to help others – through the discovery of therapies that improve the lives of people with spinal cord injuries or new ways to prevent jaundice in infants. The crux of this issue lies in the fact that uncovering information that may one day help people must be gathered from people who are living and suffering today. While research findings may one day help do good, they may also cause harm to today's research participants. For example, research participants in an AIDS study could be asked to take an experimental drug to see if it alleviates their symptoms. The participants with AIDS take on a risk (ingesting the experimental drug) in order to benefit others (information on how well the drug works) at some time in the future. Researchers must never subject research participants to more risk than necessary, be prepared to cease research if it is causing harm, and never put participants at a level of risk disproportionate to the anticipated benefits.

Justice. Particular interest has been paid lately to preventing the overburdening of some populations in order to apply research findings to other groups.

Ethical guidelines

Guidelines for the use of human subjects in research are relatively recent, with the first modern and formal efforts to protect human subjects coming after World War II. Since that time, each set of regulations and internationally adopted principles concerning research with human subjects consider the following issues to be of tantamount concern:

- Human subjects must voluntarily consent to research and be allowed to discontinue participation at any time.

- Research involving human subjects must be valuable to society and provide a reasonably expected benefit proportionate to the burden requested of the research participant.

- Research participants must be protected and safe. No research is more valuable than human well being and human life.

- Researchers must avoid harm, injury, and death of research subjects and discontinue research that might cause harm, injury, or death.

- Research must be conducted by responsible and qualified researchers.

- No population of people can be excluded from research or unfairly burdened unless there is an overwhelming reason to do so.

Medical ethics

Historically, Western medical ethics may be traced to guidelines on the duty of physicians in antiquity, such as the Hippocratic Oath, and early rabbinic and Christian teachings.

In the medieval and early modern period, the field is indebted to Muslim physicians such as Ishaq bin Ali Rahawi (who wrote the Conduct of a Physician, the first book dedicated to medical ethics) and Muhammad ibn Zakariya ar-Razi (known as Rhazes in the West), Jewish thinkers such as Maimonides, and Roman Catholic scholastic thinkers such as Thomas Aquinas.

Declaration of Helsinki

Medical ethics are based on the Declaration of Helsinki which was created by the World Medical Association to set a standard for the way human subjects are to be treated in experimentation.

This document lays out the requirements for ethical treatment of human subjects, and was drawn up as an attempt to self-regulate science. It is not a legally binding document but widely accepted as the ethical cornerstone for the treatment of human subjects.

The inception of the document was in the **early 1960's** and started as an 11 paragraph directive, the first ever of its kind. Since its inception it has had six revisions and an additional 21 paragraphs added.

The Declaration of Helsinki is named after the geographic location where the document was drawn up, Helsinki, Finland. Prior to this document the premier code of ethics was the Nuremburg Code.

The basic principles of the Declaration of Helsinki are

- Respect for the individual.
- Respect for the individual's right to make determinations and make informed decisions regarding participation in the research, both before and during the research.
- The individual's welfare always takes precedence over society or scientific needs.
- Ethical considerations must always take precedence over laws and regulations.
- If an individual is not able to grant consent

or is a minor, then consent for participation should be sought from the guardian who is acting in the individual's best interest.

Oath of Hippocrates

I SWEAR by Apollo the physician and Æsculapius, and Health, and All-heal, and all the gods and goddesses, that, according to my ability and judgment,

- I will keep this Oath and this stipulation— to reckon him who taught me this Art equally dear to me as my parents, to share my substance with him, and relieve his necessities if required; to look upon his offspring in the same footing as my own brothers, and to teach them this art, if they shall wish to learn it, without fee or stipulation; and that by precept, lecture, and every other mode of instruction,

- I will impart a knowledge of the Art to my own sons, and those of my teachers, and to disciples bound by a stipulation and oath according to the law of medicine, but to none others.

- I will follow that system of regimen which, according to my ability and judgment, I consider for the benefit of my patients, and abstain from whatever is deleterious and mischievous.

- I will give no deadly medicine to any one if asked, nor suggest any such counsel; and in like manner I will not give to a woman a pessary to produce abortion. With purity and with holiness I will pass my life and practice my Art.

- I will not cut persons labouring under the stone, but will leave this to be done by men who are practitioners of this work. Into whatever houses I enter, I will go into them for the benefit of the sick, and will abstain from every voluntary act of mischief and corruption; and, further, from the seduction of females or males, of freemen and slaves. Whatever, in connection with my professional service, or not in connection with it, I see or hear, in the life of men, which ought not to be spoken of abroad,

- I will not divulge, as reckoning that all such should be kept secret.

While I continue to keep this Oath unviolated, may it be granted to me to enjoy life and the practice of the art, respected by all men, in all times. But should I trespass and violate this Oath, may the reverse be my lot.

Physician's Oath

At the time of being admitted as a member of the medical profession:

- I solemnly pledge myself to consecrate my life to the service of humanity;
- I will give to my teachers the respect and gratitude which is their due;
- I will practice my profession with conscience and dignity; the health of my patient will be my first consideration;
- I will maintain by all the means in my power, the honor and the noble traditions of the medical profession; my colleagues will be my brothers;
- I will not permit considerations of religion, nationality, race, party politics or social standing to intervene between my duty and my patient;
- I will maintain the utmost respect for human life from the time of conception, even under threat, I will not use my medical knowledge contrary to the laws of humanity;
- I make these promises solemnly, freely and upon my honor.

The World Medical Association Declaration of Geneva (1948).

Confidentiality in research

All information collected in a research project should remain confidential

- All information about participants should be kept confidential and assigned a HIPAA compliant code
- Data should be locked away in a secure setting
- Electronic Databases should also be protected

Consent in research

Consent is defined as concurrence by a party with an action to be taken by another party.

Informed consent

- Informed consent is essential for research involving human subjects
- Informed consent should include:
- Description of the nature of the research
- Statement that the research is voluntary and participants can withdraw at any time
- Identification of risks and benefits
- Description of how confidentiality will be protected
- Description of compensation
- Description of what info researchers will share with participants
- Identification of who is responsible for research with contact information

Consent for medical procedures

Drug prescription, inoculation, surgery

Consent for acquisition and use of body fluids/tissue/organs

Donations of blood, semen, bone marrow, kidneys

Organ donations from the dead

Characteristics of voluntary informed consent

- Legal capacity
- Physical and intellectual capacity
- Informed
- Scope of actions
- Who may take such action
- For what purpose may it be taken
- Over what time-period does it apply
- Freely given
- Revocable and variable
- Delegable
- An investigator shall seek such consent only under circumstances that provide the prospective subject or the representative sufficient opportunity to consider whether or not to participate; and that minimizes the possibility of coercion or undue influence.

  (45 *CFR* 46.116)

According to CFR, the consent should be free from the following:

- Coercion
- Undue inducements
- Exploitation

Coercion

- Coercion occurs when an overt threat of harm is intentionally presented by one person to obtain compliance from another.
- Coercion does not mean:
- involuntary or under strong influence
- doing something because there are no good options

To be coercive, a subject who refuses must be made worse off than if he/she were never asked

- Requires the presence of a threat

- Perceived coercion in research can occur with
- Prisoners
- Students and staff
- Payment for research is not coercive
- Payment is an offer not a threat

Inducements

Inducements are offers that get people to do things they would not otherwise do.

Acceptable inducements:

- Usually monetary
- Medical/diagnostic services
- Results from MRI scan
- Knowledge of genetic testing
- Neuropsychological work-up for child enrolled as a "control"

Undue inducements

Excessively attractive offers that lead people to do something to which they normally would object based on risk or other fundamental value (Dickert, 2004).

Monetary inducement that alters an individual's decision-making process such that they underestimate risks;

Payments that undermine a person's capacity to exercise a free choice invalidates the consent process;

Undue inducements may prompt subjects to lie or conceal information that, if known, would disqualify them from participation.

Under 45 CFR 46.111, failure of the participant to appropriately judge risks is considered improper informed consent.

- Ambiguities in informed consent
- What is excessive?
- Reasonability of risks varies among study participants
- Impact of risk can change throughout

the study. Should the inducement also change?

- In the absence of a standard metric, IRBs vary in their assessment of risk and appropriateness of payments.

Exploitation

An exploitative transaction is one in which person A takes unfair advantage of person B (Wertheimer, 1999).

IRB's are always concerned when vulnerable individuals are paid to enroll in medical research

Solutions to avoid exploitation:

- Pay vulnerable patients more?
- Engage patient advocates?
- Exclude vulnerable populations?
- IRBs need to define what is "fair"
- Appropriate IRB member expertise

Undue inducements or exploitative subject payment can impact science.

- Unqualified subjects enrolling in FDA monitored studies
- Conceal information important for the outcome
- Less likely to report adverse events
- Skewing population
- Not disclosing participation in multiple clinical trials can confound results

The examples of exploitative research are as follows:

1. The Intrepid Guinea Pig of the Great Lakes. In 1822, accidentally shot in the gut and left with a permanent gastric fistula. William Beaumont paid him room, board, and $150 a year for use of his stomach.

2. Walter Reed's Yellow Fever Study: Paid $100 in gold for participation. $100 bonus for successful infection with yellow fever. Payable to family in the event of death.

Chapter

12

CRITICAL APPRAISAL OF RESEARCH

Critical appraisal is the procedure of warily and methodically investigating research to determine its reliability. It is an orderly practice used to recognize the strong points and limitations of a research article in order to evaluate the worth and validity of research findings. The most critical elements of a critical appraisal are an assessment of the suitability of the study design for the research question and a thorough review of the key methodological elements of this design. Other issues that also should be judged include the appropriateness of the statistical methods used and their consequent explanation, possible conflicts of interest and the significance of the research to one's own practice.

Ten questions to ask when critically appraising a research article

1. Is the study question pertinent?
2. Does the study contribute to existing knowledge?
3. What type of research question is being asked?
4. Was the study design suitable for the research question?
5. Did the methodology deal with the major sources of bias?
6. Were there any deviations from the original protocol?
7. Does the study test a stated hypothesis?
8. Were the statistical analyses carried out properly?
9. Do the data justify the conclusions?
10. Are there any conflicts of interest?

Is the study's research question pertinent?

The first query about any published research article is to determine its relevance to one's own field of work/proposed research question. Despite using rigorous methodology, a study is of modest value if it does not focus on an important topic and adds to the existing body of literature on the subject. The assessment of whether the research question is relevant is inevitably based on subjective opinion, as what might be crucial to some will be irrelevant to others. Nonetheless, the first question to ask of any research article is whether its topic is relevant to one's own field of work.

Does the study contribute to existing knowledge?

Scientific-research endeavor is often likened to 'standing on the shoulders of giants', because new ideas and knowledge are developed on the basis of previous work. Seminal research papers that make a substantive new contribution to knowledge are a relative rarity, but research that makes an incremental advance can also be of value. For example, a study might increase confidence in the validity of previous research by replicating its findings, or might enhance the ability to generalize a study by extending the original research findings to a new population of patients or clinical context.

What type of research question does the study pose?

The most fundamental task of critical appraisal is to identify the specific research question that an article addresses, as this process will determine the optimal study design and have a major bearing on the importance and relevance of the findings. A well-developed research question usually identifies three components: the group or population of patients, the studied parameter (e.g. a therapy or clinical intervention) and the outcomes of interest. In general, clinical research questions fall into two distinct categories:

Questions about the effectiveness of Treatment. These types of questions relate to whether one treatment is better than another in terms of clinical effectiveness (benefit and harm) or cost-effectiveness.

Questions about the frequency of events. Such questions refer to the incidence or prevalence of disease or other clinical phenomena, risk factors, diagnosis, prognosis or prediction of specific clinical outcomes and investigations on the quality of health care.

Was the study design appropriate for the research question?

Studies that answer questions about effectiveness have a well-established hierarchy of study designs based on the degree to which the design protects against bias. Meta-analyses of well-conducted RCTs and individual RCTs provide the most robust evidence followed by nonrandomized controlled trials, cohort studies, case-control studies, and other observational study designs. However, in

some circumstances, RCTs are either not feasible or considered ethically inappropriate. These issues are more common in non pharmaceutical trials, such as those of surgical procedures. One review of gastrointestinal surgical research found that only 40% of research questions could have been answered by an RCT, even when funding was not an impediment. Patients' preferences, the rarity of some conditions, and the absence of equipoise among surgeons proved to be the major obstacles to performing RCTs of gastrointestinal surgery in this setting. When an RCT is not feasible, the specific reasons that preclude its use will determine the type of alternate study design that can be used. Observational studies, rather than RCTs, are the most appropriate study design for research questions on the frequency of events.

The best type of study for epidemiological investigations

Did the study methods address the key potential sources of bias?

When critically appraising research, it is important to first look for biases in the study; that is, whether the findings of the study might be due to the way the study was designed and carried out, rather than reflecting the truth. It is also important to remember that no study is perfect and free from bias; it is therefore necessary to systematically check that the researchers have done all they can to minimise bias, and that any biases that might remain are not likely to be so large as to be able to account for the results observed. A study which is sufficiently free from bias is said to have **internal validity.** Bias can be attributed to chance (e.g. a random error) or to the study methods (systematic bias). Random error does not influence the results in any particular direction, but it will affect the precision of the study; by contrast, systematic bias has a direction and results in the overestimation or underestimation of the 'truth'. Systematic

Table 12.1   Purpose of investigations and study types

Purpose of investigation	Study type
Investigation of rare diseases, e.g. tumours	Case-control studies
Investigation of exposure to rare environmental factors, e.g. industrial chemicals	Cohort study in an exposed population
Investigation of exposure to multiple agents, e.g. the joint effect of oral contraceptive intake and smoking	Case-control studies
Investigation of multiple endpoints, e.g. the risk of death from various causes	Cohort studies
Estimation of incidence in exposed populations	Exclusively cohort studies
Investigation of cofactors that vary over time	Preferably cohort studies
Investigation of cause and effect	Intervention studies

biases arise from the way in which the study is conducted, be it how study participants were selected, how data was collected, or through the researchers' analysis or interpretation. Different study designs are prone to varying sources of systematic bias.

Once the study design of a given article has been identified, the researcher should use one of the available design-specific critical-appraisal checklists to decide whether the study in question is of high quality. The Critical Appraisal Skills Programme (CASP) includes such tools and the program coordinators have developed separate checklists for the appraisal of systematic reviews, RCTs, cohort studies, case-control studies, diagnostic test studies.

Systematic reviews and meta-analyses

A meticulous, standardized protocol is used in a systematic review to identify, critically appraise and synthesize all the relevant studies on a particular topic. Some systematic reviews may then proceed to a meta-analysis, in which the results from individual studies are combined statistically to produce a single pooled result. Although planning to undertake a systematic review or a meta-analysis prospectively is possible, the majority of these types of articles are retrospective and a risk of bias exists, which arises from the selection of studies and the quality of these primary sources. Publication bias, which results from the selective publication of studies with positive findings, is of particular concern, as it distorts overall perceptions of the findings on a particular topic. The QUORUM (Quality of Reporting of Meta-Analyses) statement provides a comprehensive framework for assessments of the quality of reporting in meta-analyses and systematic reviews.

Key methodological points to consider in the appraisal of systematic reviews and meta-analyses

Were all relevant studies included (i.e. was the search comprehensive, did it exclude articles on the basis of publication status or language and was the potential for publication bias assessed)? Were selected articles appraised and data extracted by two independent reviewers? Was sufficient detail provided about the primary studies, including descriptions of the patients, interventions and outcomes?

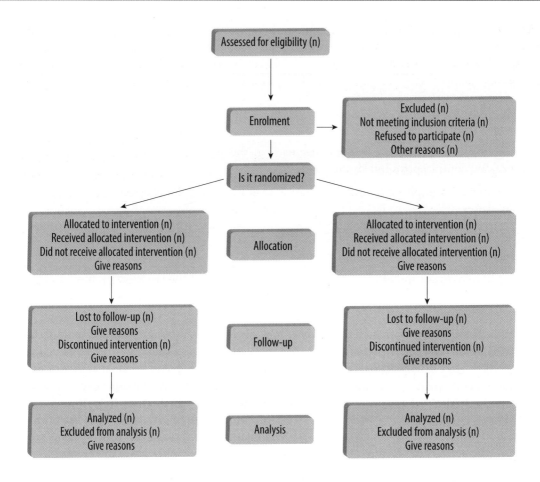

Fig. 12.1   Consolidated standards of reporting trials (CONSORT) statement flowchart for the standard reporting and appraisal of randomized controlled trials

Was the quality of the primary studies assessed? Did the researchers assess the appropriateness of combining results to calculate a summary measure?

Systematic reviews and meta-analyses are not restricted to RCTs alone. The MOOSE (Meta-Analysis of Observational Studies in Epidemiology) guidelines have been developed for meta-analyses of non-RCTs.

Randomized controlled trials

In an RCT, the random allocation of participants should ensure that treatment groups are equivalent in terms of both known and unknown confounding factors; any differences in outcomes between groups can, therefore, be ascribed to the effect of treatment. Study design alone, however, will not guard against bias if crucial aspects of the study protocol are suboptimal. The potential for selective enrollment of patients into the study can be an important source of bias if the group to which individuals will be allocated is known or can be guessed. Centralized methods of randomization, for example a computer-generated allocation, are preferable to less concealed methods, such as use of colour-coded forms or pseudo-random sequences based on medical record numbers or days of the week. Failure to conceal the allocation sequence has been shown to result in a greater distortion of the results than lack of double-blinding—another major source of bias in RCTs.

The CONSORT (Consolidated Standards of Reporting Trials) statement flow chart (Figure 1) is functionally equivalent to the QUORUM statement for systematic reviews, and provides a comprehensive tool with which to assess the standard of reporting in randomized trials. Key points to consider in the appraisal of an RCT are listed below.

Key methodological points to consider in the appraisal of randomized controlled trials

Was the process of treatment allocation truly random?

Would participants have been able to know or guess their treatment allocation?

Were participants and researchers 'blinded' to participants' treatment group?

Were outcomes assessed objectively?

Were all participants who were randomly allocated a treatment accounted for in the final analysis?

Were all participants' data analyzed in the group to which they were randomly allocated?

Cohort studies

Cohort, or longitudinal, studies involve following up two or more groups of patients to observe who develops the outcome of interest. Prospective cohort studies have been likened to natural experiments, as outcomes are measured in large groups of individuals over extended periods of time in the real world. Cohort studies can also be performed retrospectively; such studies usually involve

identifying a group of patients and following up their progress by examining records that have been collected routinely or for another purpose, such as medical data, death registry records and hospital admission databases.

The major methodological concern with cohort studies is their high potential for selection bias and confounding factors. These problems are particularly relevant when cohort studies (or non-RCTs) are used to evaluate therapeutic interventions. In this situation, the treatment that someone receives is determined by the patient's or clinician's preferences, referral patterns, current treatment paradigms or local policy. Important differences are likely to exist between patients who receive disparate treatments and these differences, rather than the treatment itself, might be responsible for the observed outcomes. Although some potential confounding factors can be measured and accounted for in the analysis, such adjustments are more difficult in retrospective than prospective studies, as data on important potential confounders might not have been collected, or might be of poor quality.

The STROBE (Strengthening the Reporting of Observational Studies in Epidemiology) statement is the corollary of the QUORUM and CONSORT statements for observational studies, including cohort, case-control and cross-sectional studies. Key methodological features to consider in the appraisal of cohort studies are listed below.

Key methodological points to consider in the appraisal of a cohort study

Is the study prospective or retrospective?

Is the cohort representative of a defined group or population?

Were all important confounding factors identified?

Were all important exposures and/or treatments, potential confounding factors and outcomes measured accurately and objectively in all members of the cohort?

Were there important losses to follow-up?

Were participants followed up for a sufficient length of time?

Case-control studies

Case-control studies are always retrospective by their very nature—the case patients are selected because they have already developed the outcome of interest (e.g. a disease). Data are then collected about factors that might have influenced this outcome, and these exposures are compared with those of a group of people who differ from the case patients only in that they have not developed the outcome of interest. Case-control studies are ideal for the investigation of risk factors when the outcome of interest is rare, as it would take too long to recruit a prospective cohort.

Major methodological difficulties with case-control studies are the selection of appropriate control individuals and the possibility of 'recall bias' (a patient's subjective interpretation of what caused their condition can alter their recall of certain events or experiences). Controls should be drawn from exactly the same population as the cases, and ideally the only difference between controls and cases should be that the controls have not developed the condition of interest. Although objective measures of possible causative factors are preferable, case-control studies often rely on participants' recall, and patients might be more likely to remember certain events or experiences than controls. Key aspects to consider when assessing a case-control study are listed below.

Key methodological points to consider in the appraisal of a case-control study

Were the cases clearly defined? Were the cases representative of a defined population?

How were the controls selected and were they drawn from the same population as the cases? Were study measures identical for cases and controls?

Were study measures objective or subjective and is recall bias likely if they were subjective?

Cross-sectional analyses

Cross-sectional studies provide a 'snapshot' in which all parameters (exposures and outcomes) are assessed at the same time; examples of cross-sectional designs include one-off surveys and audits of practice. Key methodological points to consider in the appraisal of a cross-sectional study are listed below.

Key methodological points to consider in the appraisal of a cross-sectional study

Was the study sample clearly defined?

Was a representative sample achieved (e.g. was the response rate sufficiently high)?

Were all relevant exposures, potential confounding factors and outcomes measured accurately?

Were patients with a wide range of severity of disease assessed?

Case series

Case series provide low-level evidence about therapeutic effectiveness; however, these articles are very common in medical literature. Key methodological issues to consider when assessing such articles are listed below.

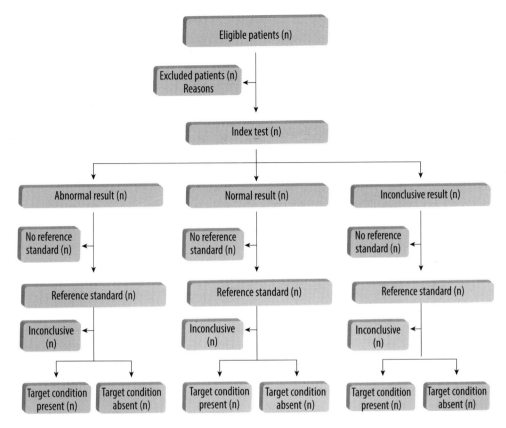

Fig.12.2   Standards for the reporting of diagnostic accuracy studies (STARD) statement flow chart for the standard reporting and appraisal of studies examining the accuracy of diagnostic tests

Key methodological points to consider in the appraisal of a case study

Were cases identified prospectively or retrospectively? Are the cases a representative sample (e.g. a consecutive series of individuals recruited from multiple centers) and similar to patients in your practice?

Were all relevant exposures, potential confounding factors and outcomes measured accurately?

Studies that assess the accuracy of diagnostic tests

These studies are usually cross-sectional in design, but possess a number of specific methodological issues that should be considered in addition to those noted above. To investigate the accuracy of a diagnostic test, it is performed on a sample of patients and the results are compared with those of a reference or gold-standard diagnostic test. The level of agreement between the investigated test and the gold-standard diagnostic test can then be reported either in terms of the sensitivity and specificity, or likelihood ratio.

The STARD (Standards for the Reporting of Diagnostic Accuracy Studies) provides a detailed flowchart (Fig.12.2) for standardized reporting and appraisal of studies that assess the accuracy of diagnostic tests. Important features to consider when appraising a study of diagnostic accuracy are listed below:

Key methodological points to consider in the appraisal of a study of diagnostic accuracy

Does the sample of patients represent the full spectrum of patients with and without the diagnosis of interest? Was there a comparison with an appropriate 'gold-standard' test?

Did all patients receive both the test under evaluation and the same 'gold-standard' test? Were the tests performed independently with blinding of assessors to the results of the 'gold-standard' test? Were the cut-offs that were used to classify patients as having a positive test result clearly described?

Was the study performed in line with the original protocol?

Deviations from the planned protocol can affect the validity or relevance of a study. One of the most common problems encountered in clinical research is the failure to recruit the planned number of participants. An estimate suggests that more than a third of RCTs recruit less than 75% of their planned sample. This deviation from the study plan not only potentially reduces the extent to which the results of the study can be generalized to real-world situations, because those who actually were recruited might be different from those who weren't for some reason, but also reduces the power of the study to demonstrate significant findings. Other differences to the original protocol might include changes to the inclusion and exclusion criteria, variation in the provided treatments or interventions, changes to the employed techniques or technologies, and changes to the duration of follow-up.

Does the study test a stated hypothesis?

A hypothesis is a clear statement of what the investigators expect the study to find

and is central to any research as it states the research question in a form that can be tested and refuted. A null hypothesis states that the findings of a study are no different to those that would have been expected to occur by chance. Statistical hypothesis testing involves calculating the probability of achieving the observed results if the null hypothesis were true. If this probability is low (conventionally less than 1:20 or $P < 0.05$), the null hypothesis is rejected and the findings are said to be 'statistically significant' at that accepted level.

Study hypotheses must crucially be identified before the study is conducted, and are usually developed from case series and cross sectional studies). If the study investigates the statistical significance of associations that were not prespecified in the original hypothesis (post-hoc analysis), such analyses are prone to false-positive findings because, at a significance level of 5% ($P = 0.05$), 1 in 20 associations tested will be significant (positive) by chance alone. When a large number of such tests are conducted some false-positive results are highly likely to occur. Another important consideration it to check that all data relevant to the stated study objectives have been reported, and that selected outcomes have not been omitted.

Where treatments for a medical condition already exist, trials can be designed to test whether a new therapy has similar efficacy to an existing one. This type of trial is called an equivalence or noninferiority trial, as its purpose is to establish that the new treatment is no worse than the existing one. Equivalence studies require that the degree of outcome difference at which the two treatments will not be considered equivalent be determined in advance. For example, researchers might decide that if the primary outcome for a new treatment is no greater than 5% worse than that of the existing treatment, the two treatments will be considered to be equivalent. Equivalence studies determine whether a new treatment is at least as good as an existing treatment so that decisions about which treatment to administer to a given patient can be made on the basis of criteria, such as cost or ease of administration.

The CONSORT statement for randomized trials has been extended to incorporate guidelines for reporting equivalence studies. A key question when appraising this type of study is whether the trial results were analyzed appropriately for an equivalence study. If a study is designed to show that a new treatment is at least as good as an existing treatment, statistical methods, for conventional testing of a hypothesis that one treatment is superior to another should not be used. Appropriate analysis of the results in an equivalence study often involves calculating confidence intervals for the treatment effect, and determining whether these limits are within the predetermined margin of noninferiority. Another key question is whether the sample size was calculated correctly for an equivalence study, as these types of study usually require a larger sample size than a corresponding superiority trial.

Were the statistical analyses performed correctly?

Assessing the appropriateness of statistical analyses can be difficult for nonstatisticians. However, all quantitative research articles should include a segment within their 'Method' section that explains the tools used in the statistical analysis and the rationale for this approach, which should be written in terms that are appropriate for the journal's readership. In particular, the approach to dealing with missing data and the statistical techniques that have been applied should be specified; patients who are lost in follow-up and missing data should be clearly identified in the 'Results' section. Original data should be presented in such a way that readers can check the statistical accuracy of the paper.

An important consideration in the statistical analysis of RCTs is whether intention-to-treat (ITT) or per-protocol analyses were conducted. According to the ITT principle, participants' data are analyzed with reference to the group to which they were randomly allocated, regardless of whether they actually received the allocated treatment. ITT analyses are preferred, because they maintain the randomization and ensure that the two treatment groups are comparable at baseline. However, if a lot of participants are nonadherant or a large proportion cross over to other treatments, an ITT analysis will be somewhat conservative and the results might be difficult to interpret. In this situation, a per-protocol analysis that includes only those patients who complied with the trial protocol can be used to supplement the ITT analysis. As pre-protocol analyses are at an increased risk of selection bias, they should not usually be used as the primary method of analysis unless a compelling reason exists to justify this approach. The CONSORT flowchart (Figure 1) enables the flow of participants and the groups used in the analysis of the trial to be clearly identified.

Do the data justify the conclusions?

The next consideration is whether the conclusions that the authors present are reasonable on the basis of the accumulated data. Sometimes an overemphasis is placed on statistically significant findings that invoke differences that are too small to be of clinical value; alternatively, some researchers might dismiss large and potentially important differences between groups that are not statistically significant, often because sample sizes were small. Other issues to be wary of are whether the authors generalized their findings to broader groups of patients or contexts than was reasonable given their study sample, and whether statistically significant associations have been misinterpreted to imply a cause and effect.

Are there any conflicts of interest?

Conflicts of interest occur when personal factors have the potential to influence professional roles or responsibilities. Members of a research team must make judgments that have the potential to affect the safety of the participants and the validity of the research findings. Researchers are in a position to decide which studies will be conducted in their unit, which patients will be invited to participate in a study and whether certain clinical occurrences should be reported as adverse events. These decisions require researchers to act with integrity and not for personal or institutional gain.

Potential financial conflicts of interest include the receipt of salary and consultation fees from the company that has sponsored the research and ownership of stocks and shares or other financial interests, such as patents related to the research. Units that recruit research participants might be paid a per-capita fee for every patient enrolled, which can be greater than the expenses involved. Many potential financial sources of conflicts of interest, such as industry funding for educational events, travel or gifts, are increasingly recognized both within the context of daily clinical practice and research. However, other potential conflicts are inherent to the research setting. An example is that medical researchers' status and future research income is dependent on the success of their research.

Identification of a potential conflict of interest is not synonymous with having an actual conflict of interest or poor research practice. Potential conflicts of interest are extremely common, and the most important questions are whether they have been recognized and how they have been dealt with. A main mechanism for dealing with potential conflicts of interest is open disclosure. In the process of critically appraising a research article, one important step is to check for a declaration about the source of funding for the study and, if a potential conflict of interest had been identified for a statement about how this conflict was managed. For example, the researchers might state specifically that the sponsoring agency had no input into the research protocol, data analysis or interpretation of the findings. Many journals now routinely require authors to declare any potential financial or other conflicts of interest when an article is submitted. The reader must then decide whether the declared factors are important and might have influenced the validity of the study's findings.

Conclusions

Critical appraisal is a systematic process through which the strengths and weaknesses of a research study can be identified. This process enables the reader to assess the study's usefulness and whether its findings are trustworthy. The most important component of critical appraisal is careful assessment of the study design; however, other steps, such as evaluation of the statistical methods used, interpretation of the findings and potential conflicts of interest are also essential. Finally, consideration of the importance of the research to one's own patients will help researchers identify the most relevant, high-quality studies available to guide their clinical practice.

Chapter 13

EVIDENCE BASED MEDICAL PRACTICE

Half of what we teach you here is wrong. Unfortunately, we do not know which half."

(Dean's address, first day of medical school)

We can certainly remember the devastating example of expert opinion gone wrong, when Dr. Benjamin Spock (1903–1998), American childcare specialist and author of the best-selling book *Baby and Child Care*, recommended that infants sleep in the prone position. Dr. Spock was considered an "expert" in child care, and his reasoning seemed quite logical—infants sleeping on their backs may be more likely to choke on vomit.

Without question, millions of healthcare workers and families began following Dr. Spock's advice, and placing babies to sleep in the prone position became standard practice. Unfortunately, no conclusive evidence existed that sleeping on the stomach was safer for infants than sleeping on the back, and as a result of this untested practice, thousands of children died as a result of sudden infant death syndrome.

Examples of untested treatments are also present in surgical literature. In this particular example, a commonly used invasive treatment was later found to provide no better outcome than less invasive treatments. Radical mastectomy, developed in the early nineteenth century by William Halsted (1852–1922), was the most common method for treating breast cancer. At the time, cancer specialists believed that breast cancer grew slowly from the tumor

outward toward the lymph nodes and that extensive removal of the affected area should cure the cancer.

Based on the belief that "more is better," the radical mastectomy involved complete removal of the affected breast and pectoralis muscles, and in the most severe cases, removal of ribs to access the lymph nodes.

Unfortunately, after widespread use of this extremely invasive procedure, survival rates did not improve. This caused cancer specialists to revise their original theory, prompting the use of lumpectomy, a less invasive surgical procedure, followed by systemic treatments such as irradiation and chemotherapy.

However, even with this new theory, many surgeons still advocated for the radical procedure, and it was not until the mid 1950s that the less invasive treatments became widely accepted.

Two American surgeons, George Crile and Bernard Fisher, were credited with bringing this issue to the forefront. While Crile was promoting the less radical procedures, Fisher and his colleagues began conducting randomized controlled trials to compare the effectiveness of radical mastectomy and lumpectomy followed by irradiation for breast cancer treatment.

After a 20-year follow-up, their results suggested that lumpectomy followed by irradiation was equally effective as radical mastectomy at treating breast cancer. If not for this new found evidence, more women would have undergone the unnecessary and highly mutilating procedure without added benefit.

After Fisher's work, additional trials were conducted in the United Kingdom, Sweden, and Italy, paving the way for the very first systematic review on breast cancer treatment. These and many other examples emphasize the importance of using valid evidence to inform clinical decisions.

Although it would be incorrect to assume that "pre–evidence-based medicine" was unscientific, modern evidence-based medicine provides a framework and cultural standard for applying the evidence, and this guidance is necessary for all specialties.

This brings us to a new paradigm for medical practice: "Evidence-based medicine", which deemphasizes

- Hunch /Gut Feeling
- Unsystematic clinical experience
- Anecdotal evidence, as sufficient grounds for clinical decision making and stresses the examination of evidence from clinical research. This paradigm shift is viewed by many physicians as another intrusion into their autonomy in taking care of patients by imposing a regimented system of care that has been viewed with skepticism and alarm.

The full-blown practice of EBM comprises five steps

1. Converting the need for information (about prevention, diagnosis, prognosis, therapy, causation, etc.) into an answerable question.

For formulating an answerable question PICO is what we need to remember. In PICO

- P stands for patient or population. We should define what are the most important characteristics of the patients about whom we are talking.

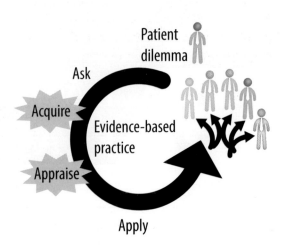

Fig.13.1   The full-blown practice of EBM comprises five steps

- I stands for intervention. What main intervention are we considering? What do we want to do with this patient?
- C stands for comparison. What is the main alternative being considered, if any?
- O stands for outcome. What are we trying to accomplish, measure, improve or affect?

Clinical scenario

A 25-years-old man presents to the emergency department with a traumatic laceration to his left index finger. The wound needs a thorough clean and will require suturing and you decide to do this using a digital nerve block technique. A colleague who has recently worked in plastic surgery suggests you to use epinephrine (1:100 000) to help with hemostasis but **you have always been told that this can cause finger necrosis and that it should never be done**. You wonder whether in fact this is true and decide to look at the evidence for yourself.

Question for this clinical scenario can be

In [adult patients with no underlying vascular compromise undergoing digital block] is [local anaesthetic with low dose epinephrine as safe as local anesthetic alone] at [achieving analgesia without causing ischaemic complications]?

After we have **converted the clinical problem into an answerable question, we generate appropriate keywords**

Key words

("Anesthesia"[MeSH] or "anesthesia, local"[MeSH]) or "nerve block"[MeSH] and "epinephrine"[MeSH] and "Fingers"[MeSH]

Search strategy

Traditional sources of information are—asking colleagues or "experts", reading textbooks, and journals. Secondary sources of reliable summarised evidence include Archimedes, Clinical Evidence and BestBets but the quality of information obtained from this source is variable. Other important sources of evidence include the online bibliographic databases which allow thousands of articles to be searched in a relatively short period of time in an increasing number of journals. Effective searches aim to maximise the potential of retrieving relevant articles within the shortest possible time. Studies have shown that, even in countries where hospitals have facilities for internet access allowing health care personnel access to a number of electronic databases, many people are not familiar with the process of carrying out efficient searches and often conduct searches which result in too few or too many articles. The ability to search following databases effectively is an important aspect of EBM.

- Cochrane library databases
- MEDLINE
- EMBASE
- CINAHL
- ARCHIMED

Search outcome

For the above scenario, Medline search using Pubmed, 16 papers retrieved of which seven were found to be relevant. There were two randomised control trials, three observational cohort studies, and two review articles. Table 13.1

Table 13.1   Relevant paper(s)

Author, date and country	Patient group	Study type (level of evidence)	Outcomes	Key results	Study weaknesses
Andrades et al. April 2003 USA	Study group (n = 21) received 2% lignocaine with 1:100 000 epinephrine and control group (n = 22) received 2% lignocaine	Randomised control trial	Pain score at one hour	Study group = 1.4, control group = 4.1 (p<0.05)	Small study
			Need for further anaesthetic dose	Study group = 4%, control group = 24% (p<0.05)	
			Duration of analgesia	Study group = 4.6 h, control group = 2.4 h (p<0.05)	
			Ischaemic damage	None	
Krunic et al. 2004 November USA	Review of all reported cases of digital gangrene associated with the use of epinephrine from National Library of Medicine	Review article	Presence of confounding factors in the reported cases	21 reported cases of digital gangrene involved the use of epinephrine. Factors such as inappropriate mixing of epinephrine, use of older agents, inappropriate use of tourniquet, use of hot soaks, infection, and large volume of injection were associated with the reported cases. No case reported epinephrine as the sole cause of gangrene.	Historical review
Wilhelmi et al. 1998 October USA	23 procedures with digital ring block using lignocaine 1% with adrenaline 1:100,000 (n=11) or 1:200,000 (n=12)	Observational cohort study	Digital-brachial pressure index (ratio of digital to brachial artery systolic blood pressures)	Mean fall of 19% in digital-brachial pressure index following the block (SD 14.6%)	The digital blood pressures were not measured at the end.

Author, date and country	Patient group	Study type (level of evidence)	Outcomes	Key results	Study weaknesses
Sylaidis et al. 1998 February UK	100 consecutive patients underwent digital ring block using lignocaine 2% with adrenaline 1:80,000	Observational cohort study	Digital-brachial pressure index (ratio of digital to brachial artery systolic blood pressures)	Mean fall of 19% in digital-brachial pressure index following the block (SD 14.6%).	The digital blood pressures were not measured at the end of procedure.
			Finger tip temperature	Mean increase of 0.8 (SD 2.3)°C following block	
			Digital artery blood flow (10 patients, duplex scanner)	Blood flow returned to normal by 1 h in all cases	
			Ischaemic damage	None	
Altinyazar et al. 2004 April Turkey	24 adults undergoing blocks in fingers or toes with 2% lignocaine and 1:100, 000 epinephrine	Observational cohort study	Digital artery blood flow at 10 min	Fall in peak systolic velocity by 60% and end diastolic velocity by 90%	
			Digital artery blood flow at 60 min (n=21)	Blood flow returned to pre-block measurement	
			Digital artery blood flow at 90 min (n=3)	Blood flow returned to pre-block measurement	

Author, date and country	Patient group	Study type (level of evidence)	Outcomes	Key results	Study weaknesses
Denkler 2001 July USA	Review of all reported cases of ischaemic digital necrosis associated with the use of epinephrine from 1880 to 2000	Review article	Presence of confounding factors in reported cases of ischaemic damage	21 out of 48 reported cases of digital gangrene involved the use of epinephrine. Confounding factors such as inappropriate concentration of epinephrine, use of older local anaesthetics, excessive volume of injection, prolonged use of tourniquet, use of hot soaks and infection were identified with all reported cases of gangrene.	
Wilhelmi et al. 2001 February USA	Study group (n = 31) had digital block using 1% lignocaine with 1:200 000 epinephrine; Control group (n = 29) had 1% lignocaine plain	Randomised control trial	Need for tourniquet	Study group = 9/31, control group = 20/29, (p<0.002)	
			Need for further anaesthetic dose	Study group = 1/31, control group = 5/29 (p = 0.098)	
			Ischaemic complications	None	

Comment(s)

Two review articles carefully examined the previously reported cases and found that no case had epinephrine as the sole cause of ischaemic complication. Two studies examined the digital perfusion using Doppler flow, and concluded that the blood flow returned to normal by one h after epinephrine injection.

Other randomised and observational studies showed longer duration of anaesthesia, better analgesia, less need for tourniquets and no ischaemic damage with the use of epinephrine. This is clearly a controversial topic as it has been emergency medicine dogma that vasoconstrictive agents should not be used in digits. However, the evidence does not support this assertion for all patients.

Clinicians may decide to use low concentration epinephrine when they feel this may help the procedure and where there is no underlying reason not to do so.

Clinical bottom line

In the absence of underlying vascular compromise, epinephrine (1:200 000 to 1:100 000) is safe to use in digital blocks along with local anaesthetics.

2. Tracking down the best evidence with which to answer that question.

What qualifies as "best evidence" differs by clinical question and rating scales. e.g Randomized controlled trials are most appropriate for therapy outcome but not appropriate when looking at the prognosis of a disease. The question in this instance is, "What will happen if we do nothing at all?" In this case, the highest evidence would come from a cohort study or a systematic review of cohort studies. A number of groups and organizations have attempted to classify and stratify high-quality versus lower-quality evidence and we know what level is appropriate to answer that question we need to search the evidence.

Evidence rating scale for therapeutic studies

Table 13.2 Level of qualifying studies evidence

I	High quality, multicentered or single-centered, cohort study validating a diagnostic test (with standard as reference) ina series of consecutive patients; or a systematic review of these studies
II	Exploratory cohort study developing dianostic criteria (with standard as reference) in a series of consecutive patients; or a systematic review of these studies
III	Diagnostic study in nonconsecutive patients (without consistently applied standard as referenc); or a systematic review of these studies
IV	Case-control study; or any of the above diagnostic studies in the absence of a universally, accepted standard
V	Expert opinion; case report or clinical example; or evidence based on physiology, bench research of "first principles

Evidence rating scale for diagnostic studies

Tale 13.3 Level of qualifying studies evidence

I	High quality, multicentered or single-centered, randomized controlled trial with adequate power; or systematic review of these studies
II	Lesser quality, randomized controlled trial; prospective cohort study; or systematic review of these studies
III	Retrospective comparative study; case-control study; or systemetic review of these studies
IV	Case series
V	Expert opinion; case report or clinical example; or evidence based on physiology, bench research of "first principles"

Table 13.4   Evidence rating scale for prognostic/risk studies

Level of qualifying studies evidence

I	High quality, multicentered or single-centered, randomized controlled trial with adequate power; or systematic review of these studies
II	Lesser quality, randomized controlled trial; prospective cohort study; or systematic review of these studies
III	Retrospective comparative study; case-control study; or systematic review of these studies
IV	Case series
V	Expert opinion; case report or clinical example; or evidence based on physiology, bench research of "first principles"

Table 13.5   Scale for grading recommendations

Grade	Descriptor	Qualifying evidence	Implications for practice
A	Strong ecommenda-tion	Level I evidence or consistent finding from multiple studies of Levels II, III or IV	Clinicians should follow a strong recommendation unless a clear and compelling rationale for an alternative approach is present.
B	Recommen-dation	Level II, III, or IV evidence and findings are generally consistent	Generally, clinicians should follow a recommendation but should remain alert to new information and sensitive to patient preferences.
C	Option	Leve II, III, or evidence, but findings are inconsistent	Clinicians should be flexible in their decision making regarding appropriate practice although they may set bounds on alternatives; patients preference should have a substantial influencing role.
D	Option	Level V: Little or no systematic empirical evidence	Clinicians should consider all options in their decision making and be alert to new published evidence that clarifies the balance of benefit versus harm; patient preference should have a substantial influencing role.

3.   **Critically appraising the evidence for:**

- Validity

- Impact

- Applicability

Many journals assign a level to the articles they publish, and authors often assign a level when submitting an abstract to conference proceedings. This allows the reader to know the level of evidence of the research, but the designated level of evidence does always guarantee the quality of the research. It is important that readers not assume that level I evidence is always the best choice or appropriate for the research question. One of the key message of evidence based medicine is "Don't believe everything you read. "In 2006, the journal Science was forced to retract two of its published articles after the research was found to be fabricated. This means that you need to evaluate or critically appraise the quality of evidence you have found

How do you critically appraise a published research?

Who? has written. Are they recognised authors? Are they affiliated to a recognised institution?

What? What are the aims and objectives?

How? Has the right research methodology been used?

When? Is it recent or seminal research?

Where? Has it been published in a recognised journal? Is it a peer reviewed journal?

Valid? Are the results valid statistically and clinically

Statistical Significance? Play of Chance (P value) conventionally taken as 0.05, Power of study conventionally taken as 80%, Sample size

Clinical significance /95% Confidence intervals? Mean ± Standard Deviation, Odds ratio confidence interval should not include 1. *Confidence interval should be narrow*

Obvious bias or conflict of interests?

What are the conclusions?

4. Integrating the critical appraisal with our clinical expertise and with our patient's unique biology, values and circumstances

Although guidelines are often criticized for being "cookbook" medicine, evidence alone cannot answer clinical questions about individual patients; clinical expertise and patient values and preferences are key elements of evidence-based medicine and are equally important in clinical decision making. Therefore, when it comes to practice guidelines, one size does not fit all, and

recommendations will not apply to every patient, yet well-developed guidelines can be helpful for developing individualized treatment plans.

5. Evaluating our effectiveness and efficiency in executing steps 1-4 and seeking ways to improve them both for next time

Conclusion

There is no way to know when our observations about complex events in nature are complete. Our knowledge is finite, but our ignorance is infinite. In medicine, we can never be certain about the consequences of our interventions, we can only narrow the area of uncertainty.

CASE HISTORY AND EXERCISE

RESEARCH STUDIES EXERCISES

Slade PD studied "Awareness of body dimensions in anorexia nervosa"

Patients suffering from anorexia nervosa usually exhibit extreme concern over their physical size and weight. This tendency, noted by many observers, has been variously interpreted. However, few studies of this phenomenon have been reported.

The objective technique for determining bodily perception is described, together with a series of studies during follow ups involving investigation of bodily perception in anorexia nervosa.

In the first study, a group of anorexia nervosa patients was compared with a group of normal female controls, results showing that, unlike the controls, the patients exhibited marked overestimation of the width of their own body. Moreover, this tendency was found not to extend to perception of physical objects.

The results showed that the overestimation of body width was less marked when the patients were required to gauge the size of a female model. In addition, they were found to be remarkably accurate in assessing physical height, both of themselves and of the model.

The effects of refeeding on the patients' tendency to see themselves as abnormally wide (and fat). The findings showed that this tendency decreased as patients put on weight.

Moreover, the degree of overestimation of body width exhibited by patients was found to bear a relationship to their progress after discharge from hospital: when this persisted after weight gain, a subsequent relapse was more likely.

The study design is:

1. **Cross-sectional**
2. **Longitudinal study**
3. Case control
4. Clinical trial

Qureshi AR studied "factors predicting malnutrition in hemodialysis patients"

The signs of protein-energy malnutrition are common in maintenance hemodialyis (HD) patients and are associated with increased morbidity and mortality. The objective was to evaluate the nutritional status and relationship between various parameters used for assessing malnutrition, and performed a study in 128 unselected patients treated with hemodialysis (HD) thrice weekly for at least two weeks. Global nutritional status was evaluated by the subjective global nutritional assessment (SGNA).

Body weight, skinfold thicknesses converted into % body fat mass (BFM), mid-arm muscle circumference, hand-grip strength and several laboratory values, including serum albumin (S_{Alb}), plasma insulin-like growth factor I (p-IGF-I), serum C-reactive protein (S_{CRP})

and plasma free amino acids, were recorded. Dose of dialysis and protein equivalence of nitrogen appearance (nPNA) were evaluated by urea kinetic modeling.

The patients were subdivided into three groups based on SGNA: group I, normal nutritional status (36%); group II, mild malnutrition (51%); and group III, moderate or (in two cases) severe malnutrition (13%). Clinical factors associated with malnutrition were: high age, presence of cardiovascular disease and diabetes mellitus. nPNA and Kt/V_{urea} were similar in the three groups. However, when normalized to desirable body weight, both were lower in groups II and III than in group I.

Anthropometric factors associated with malnutrition were low body weight, skinfold thickness, mid-arm muscle circumference (MAMC), and hand-grip strength. Biochemical factors associated with malnutrition were low serum levels of albumin and creatinine and low plasma levels of insulin-like growth factor 1 (IGF-1) and branched-chain amino acids (isoleucine, leucine and valine). The serum albumin (S_{Alb}) level was not only a predictor of nutritional status, but was independently influenced by age, sex and S_{CRP}, Plasma IGF-1 levels also reflected the presence and severity of malnutrition and appeared to be more closely associated than S_{Alb} with anthropometric and biochemical indices of somatic protein mass.

Elevated S_{CRP} (> 20 mg/liter), which mainly reflected the presence of infection/inflammation and was associated with hypoalbuminemia, was more common in malnourished patients than in patients with normal nutritional status, and also more common in elderly than in younger patients. Plasma amino acid levels, with the possible exception of the branched-chain amino acids (isoleucine, leucine, valine), seem to be poor predictors of nutritional status in hemodialysis patients.

The study design is:

1. **Cross-sectional**
2. Cohort
3. Case control
4. Clinical trial

Martin L studied "are childhood trauma exposures predictive of anxiety sensitivity in school attending youth?"

Stressful life events in adolescents have been found to be longitudinally associated with higher anxiety sensitivity (AS). A question that has not been addressed is whether AS in adolescence is associated with different childhood adversity exposures.

School attending adolescents (n=1149) completed measures of anxiety sensitivity (CASI), trait anxiety (STAI-T), childhood trauma (CTQ), depression (CES-DC), alcohol (AUDIT) and drug use (DUDIT), and resilience (CD-RISC) and coping orientation (A-COPE).

There was no significant gender difference in childhood trauma exposure, resilience levels or coping orientation. Gender differences were evident in terms of AS, trait anxiety, depression, alcohol and drug use. Depression, trait anxiety and alcohol use mediated the relationship between the amount of childhood trauma and AS and played a role in the relationship between certain childhood trauma types and AS. Neither resilience nor coping orientation had a moderating effect on the relationship between the amount of childhood trauma and AS.

Girls are at greater risk than boys for early onset anxiety disorders as girls have higher rates of AS, trait anxiety and depression despite the same rates of childhood trauma, coping orientation and resilience. Our findings, in the context of childhood trauma, underscore the influence of depression, trait anxiety and alcohol use as risk factors for the development of AS in youth. The study design is:

1. Cross-sectional
2. **Retrospective cohort**
3. Prospective cohort
4. Clinical trial

Palmer K studied "prevalence of dementia and factors associated with dementia in rural Bangladesh"

There are currently no published reports of dementia prevalence or factors associated with dementia occurrence in Bangladesh. The aims are to report the prevalence of definite and questionable dementia in rural Bangladesh, and examine factors potentially associated with dementia occurrence, including sociodemographic, clinical, social, and nutritional factors.

Methods: We used data from a population-based, study from MATLAB, in rural Bangladesh, on 471 persons aged 60+ years. Participants underwent a clinical examination including diagnosis of somatic disorders, and a structured interview including questions about sociodemographic and social factors.

Nutritional status was measured with the Mini Nutritional Assessment, and blood tests were conducted to assess a range of nutritional and clinical aspects. Age- and sex-specific dementia prevalence was calculated. Crude and adjusted logistic regression was used to examine associations between dementia and clinical, social, and nutritional factors. Dementia was diagnosed using a two-step procedure by physicians according to DSM-IV criteria. Results: The prevalence of questionable dementia was 11.5% and definite dementia was 3.6%. Dementia prevalence increased with increasing years of age (adjusted OR: 1.04; 95% CI = 1.002-1.1) and decreased with more years of education (adjusted OR: 0.8; 95% CI = 0.6-0.99). Being malnourished increased the odds of dementia almost six-fold (adjusted OR: 5.9; 95% CI = 1.3-26.3), while frequent participation in social activities was

associated with decreased odds (adjusted OR: 0.5; 95% CI = 0.2-0.9).

Conclusions: The prevalence of dementia in rural Bangladesh is similar to other countries in the South Asia region, but lower than reports from other world regions. Malnutrition is strongly associated with dementia occurrence, and is a relevant area for future research within low-income countries. The study design is:

1. **Cross-sectional**
2. Cohort
3. Case control
4. Clinical trial

Moschella PC studied "Prevalence of undiagnosed acute and chronic HIV in a lower-prevalence urban community"

The researcher estimated the seroprevalence of both acute and chronic HIV infection by using random samples from regions of the United States with low-to-moderate HIV prevalence.

Methods: This seroprevalence study consecutively enrolled patients aged 18 to 64 years within randomly selected sampling blocks in a Midwestern urban region of lower HIV prevalence in 2008 to 2009. Participants were compensated for providing a blood sample and health information. After de-identification, we assayed samples for HIV antibody and nucleic acid.

Results: There were 926 participants who consented and enrolled. Overall, prevalence of undiagnosed HIV was 0.76% (95% confidence interval [CI] = 0.30%, 1.56%). Three participants (0.32%; 95% CI = 0.09%, 0.86%) were nucleic acid-positive but antibody-negative and 4 (0.43%; 95% CI = 0.15%, 1.02%) were antibody-positive.

Conclusions. Even when the absolute prevalence is low, a considerable proportion of undetected HIV cases in an ED population are acute. Identification of acute HIV in ED settings should receive increased priority. (Am J Public Health 2014: e1-e5. doi:10.2105/ AJPH.2014.301953). The study design is:

1. **Cross-sectional**

2. Cohort

3. Case control

4. Clinical trial

Helou R studied "Occupational exposure to mineral turpentine and heavy fuels: a possible risk factor for Alzheimer's disease"

The research stated that the association between solvents and Alzheimer's disease (AD) has been the subject of several studies. Yet, only few studies have examined the various solvents separately, and the controls have rarely been monitored long enough. For these reasons and others, we believe that further studies are required.

The objective of this study was to identify solvents associated with the clinicoradiological diagnostic of AD or mixed-type dementia (MD).

A study was performed in 156 patients followed up at the Memory Diagnostic Center of Bertinot Juel Hospital (France). The inclusion criteria were known occupation(s), a Mini-Mental State Examination (MMSE) score ≥10 at the first visit, a neuropsychological evaluation performed and a diagnosis established in our Memory Diagnostic Center. The diagnostics were crossed with 9 solvents belonging to two classes of solvents. Exposure was evaluated using French national job-exposure matrices.

Certain petroleum-based solvents and fuels (i.e. mineral turpentine, diesel fuel, fuel oil and kerosene) were associated with a diagnosis of AD or MD. This association was still significant after adjustment for age, sex and education (adjusted OR: 6.5; 95% CI: 2-20).

Occupational exposure to mineral turpentine

and heavy fuels may be a risk factor for AD and MD. The study design is:

1. Cross-sectional

2. **Case control**

3. Cohort

4. Clinical trial

Gallagher JC studied "patients with carbapenem-resistant and third-generation cephalosporin-resistant Klebsiella pneumoniae bloodstream infections"

Strains of third-generation-cephalosporin-resistant K. pneumoniae (3GCRKP) and carbapenem-resistant K. pneumoniae (CRKP) are rapidly spreading. Evidence is needed to establish whether differences exist between patients at risk for 3GCKRP and CRKP bloodstream infections (BSIs), thus this study was conducted to determine if risk factors differ between these two infections.

This was a retrospective study. Inclusion criteria for cases were positive blood cultures for K. pneumoniae, first episode of BSI, age ≥ 18, and susceptibility results indicating resistance to either 3rd-generation cephalosporins (3GCRKP group) or carbapenems and cephalosporins (CRKP group). Controls were patients admitted ≥72 hours and were matched to cases by month/year and medical unit. Variables of interest were analyzed by univariate analysis and those of significance were analyzed by logistic regression.

Patients with 3GCR KP BSIs and 43 patients with CR KP BSIs were matched to 154 controls. Multivariate analyses of 3GCRKP case and control groups demonstrated that LOS >40 days (OR 17.7, 95% CI 3.7-84.3), antibiotics in the past 90 days (OR 4.3, 95% CI 1.5-11.9), and presence of a central venous catheter (OR 4.1, 95% CI 1.3-13.4) were independent risk factors. Multivariate analyses of the

CRKP case and control groups demonstrated that LOS > 40 days (OR 13.5, 95% CI 2.9-62.8) and antibiotics in the past 90 days (OR 5.9, 95% CI 1.3-26.5) were independent risk factors. The study design is:

1. Cross-sectional
2. **Case control**
3. Cohort
4. Clinical trial

Morgan CD studied "Risk factors for post-concussion syndrome in an exclusively sport-related concussion group"

Sport-related concussion (SRC) is a major public health problem. Approximately 90% of SRC are transient; however, a small percentage of patients remain symptomatic several months post-injury; a condition known as Post-Concussion Syndrome (PCS). Our objective was to identify risk factors for developing PCS in an exclusively pediatric, sport-related concussion group.

We conducted a retrospective, study within the Vanderbilt Sports Concussion Clinic (VSCC) database. Forty patients with PCS (cases) were identified and matched by age and sex to SRC control patients (1:2 matching) with documented evidence of concussion resolution within three weeks. Presenting symptoms were divided by timeframe into a 24-hour phase and 3-week phase. χ Fisher's Exact test was used for categorical variables and the Mann-Whitney U-test was used for continuous variables. Forward stepwise regression models (Pin = 0.05, Pout = 0.10) were used to identify symptoms clusters associated with PCS.

PCS was predicted by: number of previous concussions (odds ratio [OR]: 1.8; 95% confidence interval [CI]: 1.1-2.9; P = .017), pre-injury depression or anxiety (OR: 17.3; 95% CI: 2.6-116.4; P = .003), family history of depression or anxiety (OR: 2.9; 95% CI: 1.0-8.0; P = .045), family history of migraine (OR: 3.9; 95% CI: 1.53-9.80; P = .004), and neuropsychiatric symptoms within 24 hours (Exp [ß] = 0.04; 95% CI: 0.00-6.33; P = .023). Body mass index percentile did not predict PCS. According to this case-control study of risk factors for PCS in pediatric SRC, individual or family history of pre-injury depression, anxiety, or migraines portended a higher risk of developing PCS. Furthermore, increased number of previous concussions and neuropsychiatric symptoms within 24 hours predicted PCS. These results may afford practitioners greater specificity in the identification of amplified risk for PCS in young athletes. The study design is:

1. Cross-sectional
2. **Case control**
3. Cohort
4. Clinical trial

Ertunc D studied "Passive smoking is associated with lower age at menopause"

The aim of the study was to investigate the age at menopause in passive smoking women. Methods: The main outcome measure was to compare the age at menopause of secondhand smokers to non-exposed women. Results: The age at menopause in the second-hand smoking (SHS) group was significantly lower than women in the non-exposed group (47.0 + 4.7 vs 48.1 + 5.2, P = 0.002). The age at menopause had an inverse correlation with SHS, and positive correlation with mother's age at menopause in regression analyses. We further stratified women according to their smoking status. SHS women who had never smoked had significantly lower age at menopause than non-exposed women, only when the duration of exposure exceeded 20 years (46.6 + 5.6 vs 48.4 + 3.7, P = 0.008). Furthermore, never-smoked women who were exposed to > 10 cigarettes per day had significantly lower mean age at menopause than non-exposed, never-smoked women. These differences were not observed among ever-smoked women. Conclusions: Our findings suggest that earlier age at menopause should be added to the negative effects of passive smoking, in addition to increased risks for overall, cardiovascular and cancer mortality as well as an increased risk of osteoporosis. The study design is:

1. Cross-sectional
2. **Case control**
3. Cohort
4. Clinical trial

Papatoniou K studied "Colorectal cancer risk and shift work in a population in Spain (MCC-Spain)"

Epidemiological cancer studies on shift work have focused on breast cancer while evidence on other tumours is limited. We evaluated colorectal cancer risk in relation to night and rotating shift work and genetic variation, in a population based study in Spain.

1066 male and 592 female incident colorectal cancer cases and 3388 randomly selected population controls of both sexes, enrolled in 11 regions of Spain, were included. Information was collected on socio-demographic, lifestyle, medical history and other variables by face-to-face interviews. Lifetime occupational history on daily time schedule of each job, day/night/rotating shifts, light at night exposure, and duration of different jobs, was used for exposure assessment. We used unconditional logistic regression adjusting for potential confounders.

Among controls 10% of males and 4% females had ever worked full time in permanent night shifts (working between midnight and six a.m.) and 24% of males and 14% of females in rotating shifts for ≥ 1 year. Having ever performed rotating shift work was associated with an increased risk for colorectal cancer (adjusted Odds Ratio 1.33,

95% CI 1.15-1.55) compared to permanent day workers. ORs increased with cumulative years of rotating shift work and the OR for more than 30 years work 1.54 (1.22-1.94). Having ever worked in permanent night shift was not associated with colorectal cancer risk. Analysis on gene-environment interactions with genes in circadian, melatonin and sleep pathways are ongoing and will be presented.

In this large population based study we found an increase in colorectal cancer risk associated with rotating shift work. The study design is:

1. Cross-sectional
2. **Case control**
3. Cohort
4. Clinical trial

Opravil M studied "HIV-associated primary pulmonary hypertension. Swiss HIV Study"

The study was performed to assess the clinical and echocardiographic time course, prognosis, and possible etiology of HIV-associated primary pulmonary hypertension (PPH). We prospectively followed all 19 patients in whom PPH was diagnosed in our centers. Women (12 cases) and injecting drug use (16 cases) predominated; the median CD4 lymphocytes count was 83/microliter (range, 1 to 740).

Matched control subjects without PPH were identified within the Swiss HIV Study. Frozen serum samples of both groups were then reanalyzed for autoimmune parameters, neopterin, beta-2-microglobulin, and thyroid-stimulating hormone. The median follow up of the patients was 1.3 yr.

Follow-up Doppler echocardiography was available in 13 patients. The RVSP-RAP pressure gradient decreased by 3.2 mm Hg for those six patients who received antiretroviral treatment but increased by 19.0 mm Hg for untreated patients (p = 0.026). PPH was the cause of eight of 17 deaths.

The probability of surviving was significantly decreased in patients with PPH in comparison with the control subjects; the median survival was 1.3 versus 2.6 yr ($p < 0.05$). Patients with PPH had significantly higher anticardiolipin IgM, anti SS-B, and neopterin, but all other laboratory values did not differ between cases and control subjects.

In conclusion, HIV-associated PPH contributed significantly to mortality. Antiretroviral treatment may exert a beneficial effect on the pressure gradient. A possible role of an autoimmune phenomenon in the pathogenesis could not be substantiated. The study design is:

1. Cross-sectional
2. Case control
3. **Cohort**
4. Clinical trial

Chiu CY studied "sensitization to food and inhalant allergens in relation to atopic diseases in early childhood"

A correct interpretation of sensitization to common allergens is critical in determining susceptibility to allergic diseases. The aim of this study was to investigate the patterns of sensitization to food and inhalant allergens, and their relation to the development of atopic diseases in early childhood.

Children from birth through four years in the Prediction of Allergies in Taiwanese Children (PATCH) study were enrolled. Specific IgE antibody against food and inhalant allergens were measured and their association between total serum IgE levels and atopic diseases were assessed.

A total of 182 children were regular followed up at clinics for a four-year follow-up period. The prevalence of food allergen sensitization increased markedly after six months of age, reaching up to 47% at 1.5 years of age and then declined significantly to 10% in parallel with a considerable increase in the prevalence of

sensitization to inhalant allergens up to 25% at age four. Food allergen sensitization appeared to be mainly associated with the elevation of serum total IgE levels before age 2. A combined sensitization to food and inhalant allergens had an additive effect on serum IgE levels after age 2, and was significantly associated with the risk of developing atopic diseases at age 4.

Sensitization to food occurs early in life, in parallel with the rising prevalence of sensitization to inhalant allergens at older age. A combined sensitization to food and inhalant allergens not only has an additive increase in serum IgE antibody production but also increases the risk of developing allergic respiratory diseases in early childhood. The study design is:

1. Cross-sectional
2. Case control
3. **Cohort**
4. Clinical trial

Geradin P studied "Neurocognitive outcome of children exposed to perinatal mother-to-child chikungunya virus infection: The chimere study on reunion island"

Little is known about the neurocognitive outcome in children exposed to perinatal mother-to-child Chikungunya virus (p-CHIKV) infection.

The CHIMERE study compared the neurocognitive function of 33 p-CHIKV-infected children (all but one enrolled retrospectively) at around two years of age with 135 uninfected peers (all enrolled prospectively). Psychomotor development was assessed using the revised Brunet-Lezine scale, examiners blinded to infectious status. Development quotients (DQ) with subscores covering movement/posture, coordination, language, sociability skills were calculated. Predictors of global neurodevelopmental delay

(GND, DQ≤85), were investigated using multivariate Poisson regression modeling. Neuroradiologic follow-up using magnetic resonance imaging (MRI) scans was proposed for most of the children with severe forms.

The mean DQ score was 86.3 (95%CI: 81.0-91.5) in infected children compared to 100.2 (95%CI: 98.0-102.5) in uninfected peers (P<0.001). Fifty-one percent (n=17) of infected children had a GND compared to 15% (n=21) of uninfected children (P<0.001). Specific neurocognitive delays in p-CHIKV-infected children were as follows: coordination and language (57%), sociability (36%), movement/posture (27%).

After adjustment for maternal social situation, small for gestational age, and head circumference, p-CHIKV infection was found associated with GND (incidence rate ratio: 2.79, 95%CI: 1.45-5.34). Further adjustments on gestational age or breastfeeding did not change the independent effect of CHIKV infection on the neurocognitive outcome.

The mean DQ of p-CHIKV-infected children was lower in severe encephalopathic children than in non-severe children (77.6 versus 91.2, P<0.001). Of the 12 cases of CHIKV neonatal encephalopathy, five developed a microcephaly (head circumference <-2 standard deviations) and four matched the definition of cerebral palsy.

MRI scans showed severe restrictions of white matter areas, predominant in the frontal lobes in these children. The neurocognitive outcome of children exposed to perinatal mother-to-child CHIKV infection is poor. Severe CHIKV neonatal encephalopathy is associated with an even poorer outcome. The study design is:

1. Cross-sectional
2. Case control
3. **Cohort**
4. Clinical trial

Anke A studied "Functional recovery and life satisfaction in the first year after severe traumatic brain injury"

The study was done to examine the impact of demographic and acute injury-related variables on functional recovery and life satisfaction after severe traumatic brain injury (sTBI) and (2) to test whether postinjury functioning, postconcussive symptoms, emotional state, and functional improvement are related to life satisfaction. The study design was Prospective national multicenter study. Functional recovery between 3 and 12 months postinjury measured with Glasgow Outcome Scale Extended, Rivermead Postconcussion Symptoms Questionnaire, Hospital Anxiety and Depression Scale, and satisfaction with life situation.

60% of cases experienced functional improvement from 3 to 12 months postinjury. Multivariate logistic regression analysis revealed that discharge to a rehabilitation department from acute care (odds ratio [OR] = 2.14; P < .05) and fewer days with artificial ventilation (OR = 1.04; P < .05) were significantly related to improvement. At 12 months postinjury, 85% were independent in daily activities. Most participants (63%) were satisfied with their life situation. Regression analysis revealed that older age (>65 years), low education, better functional outcome, and the absence of depressive and postconcussion symptoms were significant (P < .05) predictors of life satisfaction. Functional improvement was significantly associated with emotional state but not to life satisfaction.

Following sTBI, approximately two-thirds of survivors improve between 3 and 12 months postinjury and are satisfied with their life. Direct discharge from acute care to specialized rehabilitation appears to increase functional recovery. The study design is:

1. Cross-sectionalt

2. Case control

3. **Cohort**

4. Clinical trial

Rocgue BG studied "Assessing health-related quality of life in adults with spina bifida"

The purpose of this study was to explore various aspects of health-related quality of life (HRQoL) in adults with spinal dysraphism and to compare to pediatric patients followed in a similar multi-disciplinary clinic. Researcher enrolled a prospective cohort of 31 patients from the multi-disciplinary adult spina bifida clinic. Surveys were distributed to all spina bifida patients. Data were collected using the HUI-3 health-utilities index focusing on vision, speech, hearing, dexterity, ambulation, cognition, emotions, and pain. Each participant received an overall HRQOL utility score and individual domain subscores. These were correlated with demographic and treatment variables. Scores were also compared to data from our pediatric spina bifida clinic, collected concurrently, and reported earlier. Analysis was done using SPSS Statistics (V21). There were 25 patients with myelomeningocele and six with closed spinal dysraphism. Eleven (36%) were community ambulators, and 17 (55%) were non-ambulatory. Among patients with myelomeningocele, 23 (92%) had CSF shunts in place, and three (12%) had undergone Chiari two decompression. No association was found between sex, race, age, open versus closed spinal dysraphism, insurance type, bowel or bladder continence and HRQoL. As expected, patients who were ambulatory in the community had higher ambulation QoL subscore than those who were not. History of cerebrospinal fluid shunting, Chiari two decompression, and tethered cord release also had no correlation with HRQoL scores. However, comparing HRQoL scores in adult patients to those of

159 patients followed in our pediatric clinic, we find a negative correlation between age and overall HRQoL as well as vision, emotion, pain, and ambulation subscores. Similarly, we find lower overall QoL and lower vision, emotion, and ambulation subscores in the patients from the adult clinic.

Patients followed in the adult spina bifida clinic have significantly lower HRQoL scores than those in the pediatric clinic. Other factors found to be significant in the pediatric sample, including myelomeningocele diagnosis and history of shunting, do not correlate with HRQoL in the adult clinic. The study design is:

1. Cross-sectional

2. Case control

3. **Cohort**

4. Clinical trial

Shih ST studied "Mothers After Gestational Diabetes In Australia Diabetes Prevention Program (MAGDA-DPP) post-natal intervention"

The Mothers After Gestational Diabetes in Australia Diabetes Prevention Program (MAGDA-DPP) is a randomized controlled trial (RCT) that aims to assess the effectiveness of a structured diabetes prevention intervention for women who had gestational diabetes.

The original protocol was published in Trials (http://www.trialsjournal.com/content/14/1/339). This update reports on an additional exclusion criterion and change in first eligibility screening to provide greater clarity. The new exclusion criterion "surgical or medical intervention to treat obesity" has been added to the original protocol. The risks of developing diabetes will be affected by any medical or surgical intervention as its impact on obesity will alter the outcomes being assessed by MAGDA-DPP. The screening procedures have also been updated to reflect the current recruitment operation. The first eligibility screening is now taking place either during or after pregnancy, depending on recruitment strategy. The study design is:

1. Cross-sectional

2. Case control

3. Cohort

4. **Clinical trial**

> **Fadini GP studied "Insulin-induced glucose control improves HDL cholesterol levels but not reverse cholesterol transport in type two diabetic patients"**

Type two diabetes (T2D) is characterized by low HDL cholesterol (HDL-C) and HDL dysfunction. We herein tested whether lowering HbA1c affects HDL-C and reverse cholesterol transport (RCT). Forty-two uncontrolled T2D patients initiating basal insulin were included. HbA1c, HDL-C and RCT were assessed at baseline and after six months. At baseline, HDL-C and RCT were directly correlated (r = 0.50; p < 0.001). After six months of insulin therapy, HbA1c dropped from 8.8 ± 0.16% to 7.1 ± 0.1%, while average HDL-C and RCT did not change.

Follow-up HDL-C and RCT were still correlated (r = 0.31; p = 0.033) and ΔHDL-C correlated with ΔRCT (r = 0.32; p = 0.029). ΔHbA1c correlated with ΔHDL-C (r = 0.43, p = 0.001), but not with ΔRCT. In patients with ΔHbA1c above the median value (1.3%), HDL-C (but not RCT) increased significantly. In conclusion, glucose control correlates with increased HDL-C, but not with improved RCT. Thus, persistent HDL dysfunction despite improved HbA1c and HDL-C can contribute to residual cardiovascular risk in T2D. The study design is:

1. Cross-sectional

2. Case control

3. Cohort

4. **Clinical trial**

> **Courcoulas AP studied "Surgical vs medical treatments for type two diabetes mellitus: A randomized"**

The objective of the study was to determine feasibility of a randomized clinical trial (RCT) and compare initial outcomes of bariatric surgery and a structured weight loss program for treating T2DM in participants with grades I and II obesity.

A 12-month, 3-arm RCT at a single center including 69 participants aged 25 to 55 years with a body mass index (calculated as weight in kilograms divided by height in meters squared) of 30 to 40 and T2DM. Roux-en-Y gastric bypass (RYGB), laparoscopic adjustable gastric banding (LAGB), and an intensive lifestyle weight loss intervention (LWLI).

Primary outcomes in the intention-to-treat cohort were feasibility and effectiveness measured by weight loss and improvements in glycemic control.

Of 667 potential participants who underwent screening, 69 (10.3%) were randomized. Among the randomized participants, 30 (43%) had grade I obesity, and 56 (81%) were women. Mean (SD) age was 47.3 (6.4) years and hemoglobin A1c level, 7.9% (2.0%). After randomization, seven participants (10%) refused to undergo their allocated intervention (3 RYGB, 1 LAGB, and 3 LWLI), and 1 RYGB participant was excluded for current smoking. Twenty participants underwent RYGB; 21, LAGB; and 20, LWLI, with 12-month retention rates of 90%, 86%, and 70%, respectively. In the intention-to-treat cohort with multiple imputation for missing data, RYGB participants had the greatest mean weight loss from baseline (27.0%; 95% CI, 30.8-23.3) compared with LAGB (17.3%; 95% CI, 21.1-13.5) and LWLI (10.2%; 95% CI, 14.8-5.61) (P < .001). Partial and complete remission of T2DM were 50% and 17%, respectively, in the RYGB group and 27% and 23%, respectively, in the LAGB group (P < .001 and P = .047 between groups for partial and complete remission), with no remission in the LWLI group. Significant reductions in use of antidiabetics occurred in both surgical groups. No deaths were noted. The three serious adverse events included one ulcer treated medically in the RYGB group and two rehospitalizations for dehydration in the LAGB group. The results show that RYGB was the most effective treatment, followed by LAGB for weight loss and T2DM outcomes at one year. The study design is:

1. Cross-sectional
2. Case control
3. Cohort
4. **Clinical trial**

> **Rubin M studied "Effects of rosiglitazone vs metformin on circulating osteoclast and osteogenic precursor cells in postmenopausal women with type two diabetes mellitus"**

Thiazolidinediones (TZD) are associated with increased fractures in type two diabetes mellitus (T2D). One explanation is that activation of PPAR-γ expression alters bone remodeling cells. The objective of the study was to investigate whether osteoclast and osteogenic precursor cells are altered by rosiglitazone (RSG) treatment in T2D as compared to metformin (MET).

Design: RCT of RSG or MET for 52 weeks followed by 24 weeks of MET.: Data were generated at a tertiary care center. Patients: 73 T2D postmenopausal women. Main Outcome Measures were peripheral blood mononuclear cells (PBMC) were isolated and cultured with RANK-L and stained for TRAP to measure circulating osteoclast precursors. Peripheral blood mononuclear cells were also characterized for osteogenic, endothelial and calcification markers by flow cytometry with the ligands osteocalcin (OCN), CD34 and CD 146. TRAP+ cells increased between weeks 0 and 52 (RSG: 2.9 $\pm$ 2 to 14.0 $\pm$ 3 U/L; p=0.001; MET: 3.3 $\pm$ 2 to 16.7 $\pm$ 2 U/L, p=0.001), increasing further in the RSG group after changing to MET (to 26.5 $\pm$ 5 U/L, p=0.05 vs week 52). With RSG, OCN+ cells with CD34 but without CD146 fell from week 0 to 52 (20.1 $\pm$ 1% to 15.5 $\pm$ 2%; p=0.03), remaining stable through week 76. The OCN+ cells lacking both CD34 and CD146 increased from week 0 to 52 (67.3 $\pm$ 2% to 74.4 $\pm$ 2%; p= 0.02), but returned to baseline after switching to MET.

In postmenopausal women with T2D, circulating osteoclast precursor cells increase with both RSG and MET, and increase further when switching from RSG to MET. Sub-populations of cells that may be involved in the osteogenic lineage pathway are also altered with RSG. Further work is necessary to elucidate how these changes may relate to fracture risk. The study design is:

1. Cross-sectional
2. Case control
3. Cohort
4. **Clinical trial**

> **Diele-Conwright CM studied "Evaluation of the effects of combined progressive exercise on metabolic syndrome in breast cancer survivors: rationale, design, and methods"**

Metabolic syndrome (MetS) is increasingly present in breast cancer survivors, possibly worsened by cancer-related treatments, such as chemotherapy. MetS greatly increases the risk of cardiovascular disease and diabetes, co-morbidities that could impair the survivorship experience, and possibly lead to cancer recurrence. Exercise has been shown to positively influence quality of life (QOL), physical function, muscular strength and endurance, reduce fatigue, and improve emotional well-being; however, the impact on MetS components (visceral adiposity, hyperglycemia, low serum high-density lipoprotein cholesterol, hypertriglyceridemia, and hypertension) remains largely unknown. In this trial, we aim to assess the effects of combined (aerobic and resistance) exercise on components of MetS, as well as on physical fitness and QOL, in breast cancer survivors soon after completing cancer-related treatment.

This study is investigating the effects of a 16-week supervised progressive aerobic and resistance exercise training intervention on MetS in 100 breast cancer survivors. Main inclusion criteria are histologicallyconfirmed breast cancer stage I-III, completion of chemotherapy and/or radiation within six months prior to initiation of the study, sedentary, and free from musculoskeletal disorders. The primary endpoint is MetS; secondary endpoints include: muscle strength, shoulder function, cardiorespiratory fitness, body composition, bone mineral density, and QOL. Participants randomized to the Exercise group participate in three supervised weekly exercise sessions for 16 weeks. Participants randomized to the Control group are offered the same intervention after the 16-week period of observation.

This is one of the few RCTs examining the effects of exercise on MetS in breast cancer survivors. Results contribute a better understanding of metabolic disease-related effects of resistance and aerobic exercise training and inform intervention programs that will optimally improve physiological and psychosocial health during cancer survivorship, and that are ultimately aimed at improving prognosis. The study design is:

1. Cross-sectional

2. Case control

3. Cohort

4. **Clinical trial**

O'Neill TJ studied "The effect of HIV-Hepatitis C co-infection on bone mineral density and fracture"

There is a variable body of evidence on adverse bone outcomes in HIV patients co-infected with the hepatitis C virus (HCV). The researcher examined the association of HIV/HCV co-infection on osteoporosis or osteopenia (reduced bone mineral density; BMD) and fracture on systematic review and random effects meta-analyses.

A systematic literature search was conducted for articles published in English up to one April 2013. All studies reporting either BMD (g/cm2, or as a T-score) or incident fractures in HIV/HCV co-infected patients compared to either HIV mono-infected or HIV/HCV uninfected/seronegative controls were included. Random effects meta-analyses estimated the pooled odds ratio (OR) and the relative risk (RR) and associated 95% confidence intervals (CI).

Thirteen eligible publications (BMD N=6; Fracture=7) of 2,064 identified were included with a total of 427,352 subjects. No publications reported data on HCV mono-infected controls. Meta-analysis of cross-sectional studies confirmed that low bone mineral density was increasingly prevalent among co-infected patients compared to HIV mono-infected controls (pooled OR 1.98, 95% CI 1.18, 3.31) but not those uninfected (pooled OR 1.47, 95% CI 0.78, 2.78). Significant association between co-infection and fracture was found compared to HIV mono-infected from cohort and case-control studies (pooled RR 1.57, 95% CI 1.33, 1.86) and compared to HIV/HCV uninfected from cohort (pooled RR 2.46, 95% CI 1.03, 3.88) and cross-sectional studies (pooled OR 2.30, 95% CI 2.09, 2.23).

The associations of co-infection with prevalent low BMD and risk of fracture are confirmed in this meta-analysis. Although the mechanisms of HIV/HCV co-infection's effect on BMD and fracture are not well understood, there is evidence to suggest that adverse outcomes among HIV/HCV co-infected patients are substantial. The study design is:

1. Cross-sectional
2. Case control
3. Cohort
4. **Meta-analysis**

Cao S studied "Herpes simplex virus type two and the risk of cervical cancer"

The objective was to assess whether herpes simplex virus type 2 (HSV-2) infection has an effect on the risk of cervical cancer. A systematic literature search of PubMed, Embase, Web of Science, and Scopus from their inception through July 2013, was conducted and reference lists of retrieved articles were reviewed. Information on the characteristics of the included studies, risk estimates, and control for possible confounding factors was extracted independently by two investigators. A random effects model was used to calculate the pooled risk estimates.

Sixteen articles with 20 studies (14 case control and six longitudinal) involving 3,337 patients with cervical cancer were included. Compared with individuals who did not experience HSV-2 infection, the pooled ORs of cervical cancer for individuals with HSV-2 infection were 1.37 (95 % CI 1.12-1.69) for traditional case-control studies and 1.04 (95 % CI 0.82-1.31) for prospective or retrospective nested case-control studies. The existing observational epidemiological evidence do not support a harmful effect of HSV-2 infection on cervical cancer. The study design is:

1. Cross-sectional
2. Case control
3. Cohort
4. **Meta-analysis**

Fong FM studied "Maternal genotype and severe preeclampsia: A huge review"

Severe preeclampsia is a common cause of maternal and perinatal morbidity worldwide. The disease clusters in families; however, individual genetic studies have produced inconsistent results. Researcher conducted a review to examine relationships between maternal genotype and severe preeclampsia. Researcher searched the MEDLINE and Embase databases for prospective and retrospective cohort and case-control studies reporting associations between genes and severe preeclampsia. Four reviewers independently undertook study selection, quality assessment, and data extraction. Researcher performed random-effects meta-analyses by genotype and predefined functional gene group (thrombophilic, vasoactive, metabolic, immune, and cell signalling). Fifty-seven studies evaluated 50 genotypes in 5,049 cases and 16,989 controls. Meta-analysis showed a higher risk of severe preeclampsia with coagulation factor V gene (proaccelerin, labile factor) (F5) polymorphism rs6025 (odds ratio = 1.90, 95% confidence interval: 1.42, 2.54; 23 studies, $I^2 = 29\%$), coagulation factor II (thrombin) gene (F2) mutation G20210A (rs1799963) (odds ratio = 2.01, 95% confidence interval: 1.14, 3.55, 9 studies, $I^2 = 0\%$), leptin receptor gene (LEPR) polymorphism rs1137100 (odds ratio = 1.75, 95% confidence interval: 1.15, 2.65; 2 studies, $I^2 = 0\%$), and the thrombophilic gene group (odds ratio = 1.87, 95% confidence interval: 1.43, 2.45, $I^2 = 27\%$). There were no associations with other gene groups. There was moderate heterogeneity between studies and potential for bias from poor-quality genotyping and inconsistent definition of phenotype. Further studies with robust methods should investigate genetic factors that might potentially be used to stratify pregnancies according to risk of complications. The study design is:

1. Cross-sectional

2. Case control

3. Cohort

4. **Meta-analysis**

> **Li JW studied "Can serum levels of alkaline phosphatase and phosphate predict cardiovascular diseases and total mortality in individuals with preserved renal function?"**

It is demonstrated that elevated serum levels of alkaline phosphatase (ALP) and phosphate indicate higher risks of cardiovascular disease (CVD) and total mortality in a population with chronic kidney disease (CKD), but it remains unclear whether this association exists in people with normal or preserved renal function.

Clinical trials were searched from Embase and PubMed from inception to December 2013, using the keywords "ALP", "phosphate", "CVD", "mortality" and so on, and finally 24 trials with a total of 147,634 patients were included in this study. Dose-response and semi-parametric meta-analyses were performed.

A linear association of serum levels of ALP and phosphate with risks of coronary heart disease (CHD) events, CVD events and deaths was identified. The relative risk (RR)of ALP for CVD deaths was 1.02 (95% confidence interval [CI], 1.01-1.04). The RR of phosphate for CVD deaths and events was 1.05 (95% CI, 1.02-1.09) and 1.04 (95% CI: 1.03-1.06), respectively. A non-linear association of ALP and phosphate with total mortality was identified.

Compared with the reference category of ALP and phosphate, the pooled RR of ALP for total mortality was 1.57 (95% CI, 1.27-1.95) for the high ALP group, while the RR of phosphate for total mortality was 1.33 (95% CI, 1.21-1.46) for the high phosphate group. It

was observed in subgroup analysis that higher levels of serum ALP and phosphate seemed to indicate a higher mortality rate in diabetic patients and those having previous CVD.

The higher total mortality rate was more obvious in the men and Asians with high ALP. A non-linear relationship exists between serum levels of ALP and phosphate and risk of total mortality. There appears to be a positive association of serum levels of ALP/phosphate with total mortality in people with normal or preserved renal function, while the relationship between ALP and CVD is still ambiguous. The study design is:

1. Cross-sectional

2. Case control

3. Cohort

4. **Meta-analysis**

> **Kim G studied "Overview and recent trends of systematic reviews and meta-analyses in hepatology"**

A systematic review (SR) is a research methodology that involves a comprehensive search for and analysis of relevant studies on a specific topic. A strict and objective research process is conducted that comprises a systematic and comprehensive literature search in accordance with predetermined inclusion/exclusion criteria, and an assessment of the risk of bias of the selected literature. SRs require a multidisciplinary approach that necessitates cooperation with clinical experts, methodologists, other experts, and statisticians. Meta-analysis (MA) is a statistical method of quantitatively synthesizing data, where possible, from the primary literature selected for the SR. Review articles differ from SRs in that they lack a systematic methodology such as a literature search, selection of studies according to strict criteria, assessment of risk bias, and synthesis of the study results. The importance of evidence-based medicine (EBM) in the decision-making for public policy has recently been increasing thanks to the realization that it should be based on scientific research data. SRs and MAs are essential for EBM strategy and evidence-based clinical practice guidelines. This review addresses the current trends in SRs and MAs in the field of hepatology via a search of recently published articles in the Cochrane Library and Ovid-MEDLINE.

The study design is:

1. Cross-sectional
2. Case control
3. Cohort
4. **Systematic review**

Buiedo BM studied "Current evidence for spinal opioid selection in postoperative pain"

Spinal opioid administration is an excellent option to separate the desirable analgesic effects of opioids from their expected dose-limiting side effects to improve post-operative analgesia. Therefore, physicians must better identify either specific opioids or adequate doses and routes of administration that result in a mainly spinal site of action rather than a cerebral analgesic one. The purpose of this topical review is to describe current available clinical evidence to determine what opioids reach high enough concentrations to produce spinally selective analgesia when given by epidural or intrathecal routes and also to make recommendations regarding their rational and safety use for the best management of postoperative pain. To this end, a search of Medline/Embase was conducted to identify all articles published up to December 2013, on this topic. Recent advances in spinal opioid bioavailability, based on both animals and humans trials support the theory that spinal opioid bioavailability is inversely proportional to the drug lipid solubility, which is higher in hydrophilic opioids like morphine, diamorphine and hydromorphone

than lipophilic ones like alfentanil, fentanyl and sufentanil.

Results obtained RTCs is considered to be the 'highest' level and support their use. The study design is:

1. Cross-sectional
2. Case control
3. Cohort
4. **Meta-analysis**

Kilbourne et al. (1983) investigated an epidemic in Spain involving multiple organ systems

Patients presented with cough, dyspnea, plueritic chest pain, headache, fever, and bilateral pulmonary infiltrates. Although an infectious agent was suspected, a strong association with cooking oil sold as olive oil but containing a high proportion of rape seed oil was detected. Epidemiological studies found that virtually all patients had ingested such oil but unaffected persons had rarely done so.

1. Descriptive
2. Cohort
3. **Case control**
4. Clinical trial

Kuntson et al. (1981) treated wounds and burns using granulated sugar combined with povidone-iodine (PI)

The study was undertaken from January 1976, to August 1980. During that time, 759 patients were treated. Of these, 154 were treated with the standard therapy and the remaining 605 were treated with sugar and PI. Uniformity in treatment and judgment regarding the healing process were enhanced by using three physician-investigators to oversee the process and by documenting wound healing. The investigators reported that a much lower percentage of patients treated with the sugar- PI mixture required skin grafting than those given standard treatment

1. Descriptive
2. Cohort
3. Case control
4. **Clinical trial**

Coldiz et al (1987) reported on the relationship between menopause and the risk of coronary heart disease in women

Subjects in the study were selected from 130,000 married female registered nurses aged 30-55. the investigators identified 116,000 of these women who were pre-menopausal and did not have a diagnosis of coronary heart diseases at the beginning of the study. The investigators were interested in determining that whether the influence of menopause status is altered by the use of postmenopausal estrogen.

The original survey provided information on the subject age, parental history of myocardial infractions, smoking status, height, weight, use of oral contraceptives or postmenopausal hormones and history of myocardial infraction or angina pectoris, diabetes, hypertension or high serum cholesterol levels. Follow-up surveys were done in 1978, 1980 and 1982.

1. Descriptive
2. **Cohort**
3. Case control
4. Clinical trial

Research evaluation proforma

Name Researcher:

Evaluation for format

Title	Yes	No	Comments
Reflects the objective of the study	√		
Does not contain any abbreviations	√		
Introduction			
1. Topic adequately introduced		√	
2. Relevant to the objectives			
3. Relatively new references quoted			
4. Rationale given			
5. Maximum 500 words			
Objective			
Objective stated according to SMART criteria identifying the outcome variables	√		
Appropriate operational definition given	√		
Hypothesis appropriately stated for all interventional, cohort, case control and comparative cross sectional studies	√		
Material and Methods			
Setting of the study mentioned	√		
Duration of the study mentioned		√	
Study design suitable for the objectives		√	

Sampling technique appropriate		√	
Inclusion criteria appropriate	√		
Exclusion criteria appropriate		√	
Sample size appropriate		√	
Data collection procedure			
Steps of data collection procedure in proper sequence		√	
Randomization/Blinding mentioned if required			
Confounding variables controlled		√	
Bias, if any controlled		√	
Proforma appropriate		√	
Statistical Review			
Variables under study mentioned		√	
Statistics appropriate according to the variables		√	
Statistical software mentioned	√		
Data analysis relevant to objectives		√	
Scheduling/Phasing given			
Bibliography			
References in Vancouver style		√	
Recent references mentioned (last five years)	√		
All references can be authenticated			

Evaluation for contribution to the field

Novelty	Yes	No	Comments
No work has ever been done previously anywhere		√	
Similar work reported from other countries in last five years	√		
Similar work not done in Pakistan in last five years		√	
Some studies available in Pakistan	√		
Well reported in local literature	√		
Potential for capacity building	√		
Multidisciplinary	√		
Contribution towards public benefit	√		
Contribution towards medical knowledge	√		

Decision

To be forwarded to IRB ☐

To be sent back to the Board of Studies √

Evaluated by
